AFFIRMATIVE ACTION IN MEDICINE

Affirmative Action

IN MEDICINE

Improving Health Care for Everyone

JAMES L. CURTIS, M.D.

THE UNIVERSITY OF MICHIGAN PRESS
Ann Arbor

TO VIOLA WERTHEIM BERNARD, M.D.,
A LEADER IN THE DESEGREGATION OF
POSTGRADUATE TRAINING IN PSYCHIATRY
AND PSYCHOANALYSIS

2006   2005   2004   2003   4   3   2   1

A CIP catalog record for this book is available from the British Library.

Library of Congress Cataloging-in-Publication Data

Curtis, James L., 1922–
    Affirmative action in medicine : improving health care for
everyone / James L. Curtis.
        p. ; cm.
    Includes bibliographical references and index.
    ISBN 0-472-11298-8 (cloth : alk. paper)
        1. Social medicine.   2. Affirmative action programs.   3. Right to health care.
    4. Social justice. [DNLM: 1. Health Manpower—United States.   2. Physicians—supply
    & distribution—United States.   3. Blacks—United States.   4. Cultural Diversity—
    United States.   5. Education, Medical—trends—United States.   6. Schools, Medical—
    United States. W 76 C979a 2002]   I. Title.
    RA427 .C75 2002
    362.1'0973—dc21   2002014102

CONTENTS

TABLES

PREFACE

In *Blacks, Medical Schools, and Society*, published more than three decades ago, I heralded the beginning of affirmative action to increase the enrollment of Blacks in American medical schools. Then in 1980 I wrote a book-length progress report evaluating the outcomes of affirmative action in the first decade of this nationwide initiative. That review outlined the still-formidable racial barriers separating Black people from medical education, including postgraduate training to become specialists. One result of the small number of Black physicians and specialists was inequitable treatment for Black patients in hospitals and doctors' offices. In 1980, the time I reviewed the status of Black medical education, many racial barriers were coming down faster than ever before, but affirmative action programs were coming under severe political and legal attacks.

In this book, I present a thirty-year progress report on affirmative action in medicine, defined in a comprehensive manner. This includes a review of the medical careers of approximately two thousand minority students who were admitted to the nation's medical schools beginning in 1969, who graduated through 1977, and who were in practice as of 1994. Their careers are compared to approximately two thousand randomly selected non-minority medical school graduates during those same years. These two samples provide a view of medical schools around the country, and of the much larger number of postgraduate training programs the two groups entered before setting up their still larger array of practices throughout the United States.

The reader should know that I am Black, and that for a twelve-year period from 1968 to 1980 I was associate dean and associate professor of psychiatry at Cornell University Medical College. I was recruited to join the administration and faculty for the express purpose of leading the medical school's new minority admissions program. During those years I served not only on the admissions committee but also on all committees relating to student affairs, including the internship advisory committee, as well as the governing faculty councils, and I subsequently became responsible for affirmative action programs aimed at faculty recruitment.

While I was at Cornell I also served as one of the five members of the New York City Board of Health, and on several New York State advisory committees and task forces dealing with health care delivery and health manpower policies. In the course of that work I became more acutely aware that health care policies, often appropriate for the population as a whole, sometimes ran directly counter to the health and welfare best interests of minority communities. My presence in, and contributions to, those deliberations sometimes helped to formulate more equitable and complete recommendations.

From 1982 until the beginning of 2000, I served as director of psychiatry of Harlem Hospital Center and clinical professor of psychiatry at Columbia University College of Physicians and Surgeons. My aim on assuming that position was to help develop a first-rate mental health and substance abuse service in the central Harlem community. My work was enhanced by my membership on several important advisory committees at local and state levels, such as the New York State Multicultural Advisory Committee, the Mental Health Services Council that approves all service programs, and the Mental Health Planning and Advisory Committee, charged with advising the commissioner of mental health and the governor on service programs that would best serve all citizens of the state.

Harlem Hospital Center is one of the larger units of the New York City Health and Hospitals Corporation, which consists of eleven acute care general hospitals, in various and often very different neighborhoods throughout the city, and a number of large primary health care centers. It is one of the teaching hospitals affiliated with Columbia University, and since the mid-1960s medical staff have been members of the Columbia faculty responsible for the quality of service and for postgraduate residency training programs. My retirement at the end of 1999 provided me with the necessary time to complete this thirty-year progress report evaluating the effectiveness of affirmative action in medicine.

During the 1920s and 1930s, Dr. Franklin McLean, dean of the University of Chicago Medical School, became increasingly concerned about the serious racial injustice and unfairness that prevented Blacks from receiving first-class medical education and training and first-class health care, and he realized that these objectives are linked.

With the help of the Julius Rosenwald Fund, Dr. McLean's first program priority was to form a group of leading Black and White physicians in Chicago, who then transformed Provident Hospital, a hospital in the Black ghetto, into a university-affiliated teaching hospital offering first-rate postgraduate training programs to Blacks. The program gradually expanded to promote the acceptance of Black physicians into previously racially segregated postgraduate training programs in the other teaching hospitals in Chicago. Later the vision and mission of the program expanded nationally, and in 1952 it became the National Medical Fellowships, Incorporated. In 1946, when I graduated from the University of Michigan Medical School, fewer than one hundred of the four thousand Black physicians in the United States had been trained as specialists in any branch of medicine.

In 1949 I was one of the first physicians selected for a National Medical Fellowship (NMF), which financed my postgraduate training in psychiatry and psychoanalysis. I was awarded a stipend that paid for my psychoanalytic training, which required five visits a week for several years. I had chosen to specialize in psychiatry because there were only eight Black board-certified psychiatrists in the late 1940s. Further, none had completed psychoanalytic training and certification until I was certified in that field in 1954. Shortly after the end of World War II a small group of American psychiatrists formed an ad hoc committee to desegregate postgraduate training in psychiatry. The group consisted of Dr. Helen McLean, wife of Franklin McLean and a member of the faculty of the Chicago Psychoanalytic Institute, Drs. Karl and William Menninger of the Menninger Clinic, Dr. Howard Potter, head of psychiatry and dean, State University of New York (Downstate) and Dr. Charlotte Babcock, a psychoanalyst and psychiatrist from the University of Pittsburgh who also was a member of the National Medical Fellowships Board. Dr. Viola Bernard, who was my training analyst for more than three years, had been a principal member of this group of psychiatrists and psychoanalysts who opened up our field for Black physicians.

When Dr. McLean's health began to fail in the late 1960s, leadership of NMF passed to Dr. Irving P. Graef, an internist in New York City and faculty member of the New York University Medical School. During Dr. Graef's leadership, the principal program priority of NMF progressed beyond the opening up of postgraduate training opportunity and encompassed the admission of minority students to medical schools. Beginning in 1959 and for the next ten years, the Alfred Sloan Jr. Foundation provided scholarships to a small group of very able Black medical school applicants, selected for their scholastic ability, to attend one of the predominantly White medical schools, with the aim of showing by their excellent work that it was time to desegregate medical education in this country. By the early 1970s, NMF again changed its mission and took on the responsibility of providing financial aid, not only for a few high achievers, but for all Blacks who had been accepted at any U.S. medical school. Undoubtedly this provided a major incentive for the medical schools to accept greater numbers of minority students. Indeed, NMF in 1970 began to provide financial aid not only to Blacks, but to other underrepresented minority groups such as Mexican Americans, Puerto Ricans from the U.S. mainland, and Native Americans.

When the Association of American Medical Colleges and all the leading health care and other institutions announced their endorsement of affirmative action admissions of minorities in 1970, NMF played a central role. National Medical Fellowships raised funds from a number of leading foundations and corporations to provide financial aid for a group of students who came from families who would not have been able to pay their way. Dr. Graef was succeeded for several years by Robert Stepto, a Black physician and a former NMF Fellow who had also earned a Ph.D., preparing him for a career in academic medicine. During the 1970s I served not only as a member of the NMF board, but also as its chairman for several years.

In 1968–69, Black Americans were 2.2 percent of the 35.8 thousand total medical school enrollment; Native Americans were 0.02 percent, Mexican Americans 0.16 percent, and mainland Puerto Ricans 0.01 percent. Of the 2.4 percent total underrepresented minority enrollment, 58 percent of the Black enrollees were students at Howard and Meharry, the two predominantly Black medical schools. By 1975–76, Black Americans were 6.2 percent of the much larger 55.8 thousand total U.S. medical school enrollment; Native Americans were 0.3 percent, Mexican Americans 1.3 percent, and mainland Puerto Ricans 0.4 percent. Of this total underrepresented minority enrollment of 8.1 percent, only 12.45 percent were matriculants of Howard and Meharry. Medical education in our nation for the first time had become essentially racially desegregated. This accomplishment owes much to a few men and women who felt a strong personal dedication to the cause of our common humanity. (All data in this paragraph are from table 2 in Odegaard 1977 [31]. The source of the information in the table is Association of American Medical Colleges enrollment data.)

American medicine has indeed changed, mirroring changes in our society at large, and these changes have been both faster and more far reaching than is commonly recognized. In one of the last conversations I had with Dr. Graef before his death in 1979, he recalled the changes he had lived through as a Jew. He reminisced that during the 1920s, when he was a medical student at Cornell, Cornell admitted no more than five Jews a year. When he graduated in 1926, Cornell's teaching hospital, the New York Hospital, was not receptive to Jewish applicants for postgraduate training, and that was why he went to Chicago, where he became a friend of Dr. Franklin McLean, for training. Anti-Semitic bigotry of that kind was widespread in those years. Dr. Graef went on to say that prior to World War II, there was hardly a medical school in the nation that had a Jew as head of the department of medicine, but within three decades, by 1979, there was hardly a medical school where the head of medicine was not a Jew.

As we shall note, but without major emphasis in this book, the increased enrollment of minority groups in American medical schools in this past decade has occurred in tandem with a still more dramatic fourfold increase in the representation of women. In so many ways things have changed, but as I relate in some detail in this book, it can also be said that the more things change, the more they stay the same. Much remains to be done. Future prospects for improvements in health status, physician education and training opportunity, and health care services for Black Americans are embedded in the structure and function of American society. I continue to believe that there is a favorable prospect for constructive change.

James L. Curtis, M.D.

ACKNOWLEDGMENTS

Minority programs at Cornell University Medical College enjoyed full support of the Cornell University Medical College, from President Dale Corson to President Frank Rhodes, from Deans Robert Buchanan, Theodore Cooper, and Thomas Meikle to Drs. Hugh Luckey and David Thompson, who succeeded him as executive director of the New York Hospital. I also enjoyed the close support of other associate deans at the Medical College, among them Drs. Charles Santos-Buch, John Ribble, and Susan Kline.

A number of people assisted me in writing this book, especially by making available to me data that were not easily obtained. My thanks go to Dario Prieto and Juel Hodge-Jones of the Association of American Medical Colleges, Office of Minority Affairs during the 1970s; to Leon Johnson and William Cadbury Jr. of National Medical Fellowships; and to Dr. Wilbert Jordan, who shared questionnaire data collected in his studies of minority internship choices. To Jean C. Lee, then assistant director of research for the Division of Biostatistics of the New York City Health Department, I am indebted for assistance in the compilation of data for chapter 6. To Dr. John Graettinger, then vice-president of the National Internship and Residency Matching Plan, I am particularly grateful for assistance and guidance on the use of data allowing me to study comparable samples of minority and nonminority internship candidates. These data could not have been handled without computer assistance provided by Susan Widing of the Cornell University Medical College Computer Laboratory. Ms. Widing trained teams of five students each who assisted me in preparing and analyzing this information in the summers of 1974, 1975, 1976, and 1977, and my gratitude is very great to them all: Frank Richards, Rupa Redding, Donald Wallerson, Patricia Samuels, and Irma Matos; Rafael Soltren, Edward James, Anthony Cannon, Gary Butts, and Edward Alexander; Magda Barini-Garcia, Roy Cobb, Hans Gerdes, Christopher Hannum, and Gerald Hoke; Blaine Morton, Saadia Griffith, Anthony DeMond, James Ramseur, and Carl McDougal.

Guidance and assistance on statistical analysis and presentation of data in those years were provided by Dr. Valerie Mike, head of the Biostatistics Laboratory, Sloan-Kettering Institute for Cancer Research, and to Dr. Ying Wang and Ms. Cynthia Kosloff, statisticians on her staff. To Dr. Valerie Miké, who was professor of biostatistics in public health of the Cornell University Medical College, I am additionally indebted for her careful reading of the entire 1980 manuscript and several discussions that led to the correction of several errors and additional data collection.

Among other friends and colleagues who read parts I and II of the book in whole or part as it was being written, and whose helpful encouragement, suggestions, and comments were gratefully received, were the following: Dr. Marion Mann, former dean of the Howard University College of Medicine; Professor Doris Schwartz, former professor of public health nursing at Cornell; Dr. Walsh McDermott, then special adviser to the president of the Robert Wood Johnson Foundation; Dr. George Reader, who succeeded Dr. McDermott as chairman of the Department of Public Health at Cornell; and Dr. Thomas Meikle, then dean of Cornell University Medical College.

Several consultants were of vital importance in helping to write part III, the thirty-year progress report; and in organizing the entire manuscript, Elizabeth Kramer provided excellent editorial suggestions. Dr. E. Joel Millman provided statistical advice and analyses of the extensive data presented in chapter 7, and gave helpful suggestions on the whole manuscript. I am indebted to colleagues who critically reviewed the manuscript: Dr. Bruce Ballard, who succeeded me as associate dean at Cornell and who gave information on both the twenty- and thirty-year affirmative action program at Cornell, and Drs. Alfred Gellhorn, Bertrand Bell, Katherine Lobach, and Barry Bateman. Ms. Barbara M. Simpson provided expert and devoted secretarial assistance, as did Mr. Frank Passic for a period of time.

To my wife, Vivian, I acknowledge the considerable assistance and encouragement that made this work possible. She was for many years director of social work for the Kings County Hospital in Brooklyn, one of the nation's largest municipal hospitals. Many of my ideas were formed in the course of our discussions of the public and private hospital systems in New York, and our discussions of the parallel problems of professional advancement of Blacks in the fields of social work and medicine.

James L. Curtis, M.D.

INTRODUCTION

This book is about affirmative action in undergraduate and postgraduate medical education, a significant part of my life's work. Affirmative action in medicine is defined comprehensively, covering not only the equitable opportunity to be admitted to the best medical schools and postgraduate training programs, but also the equitable provision of health care. Major emphasis is placed here on the serious differentials in health status between Blacks (or Afro-Americans) and Whites or (Euro-Americans), because the social, political, and economic contrast between these two groups has been one of the defining issues of our national history. As a Black physician and medical educator, I maintain that the persistence of a system of color caste consigns our people to a subordinate social role that is a handicap separate from the poverty Black people also endure.

More equitable recruitment of competent Black physicians can help meet the needs of Blacks who currently receive poor care. In 1970 the Association of American Medical Colleges (AAMC) and the medical establishment of our nation supported an affirmative action goal of admitting 12 percent minority students to our nation's medical schools by 1975. This effort fell short, achieving only 10 percent by that date. Again in 1990, the AAMC announced the aim of enrolling three thousand underrepresented minority students by the year 2000, but that effort failed by almost one thousand students. The reasons are clear. Medical schools quite properly will admit only those who are almost certain to graduate, and the substandard educational opportunity available to Black youngsters constricts the pipeline. Blacks become physicians at about one-half the rate of other ethnic groups (Petersdorf et al. 1990; Johnson 1998).

My outlook for future amelioration of this disparity is more optimistic than might be supposed, perhaps because of my personal life history. Both of my parents were born in the 1890s in a small farming village in Georgia. Following his military service in World War I, my father moved to Michigan in 1921 in response to labor recruiters seeking workers for the booming automobile industry. I was nine months old when, in 1922, my mother and I joined him in Albion, Michigan. Fortunately Albion, then a town of about ten thousand, was both a small factory town and the home of Albion College, one of the best small schools in the Midwest. Fortunately, opportunities came my way. I grew up in a strong, albeit racially segregated, Black community where the men all worked and supported their families. I had the further advantage of excellent schooling, which led to Albion College and then to the University of Michigan Medical School, from which I graduated in 1946. My career has been in academic medicine, the last position being that of director of psychiatry at Harlem Hospital Center and clinical professor of psychiatry at the Columbia University College of Physicians and Surgeons in New York City, from which I retired after eighteen years at the end of 1999. My story demonstrates what one can achieve in this country, given the right combination of ability, a strong support system, and just plain luck. In other words, I have had the good fortune of living and struggling with the troublesome problems that are detailed in this book.

The state of health for Black Americans is a national problem; the overall mortality rate for Blacks is 1.6 times the rate for Whites. In 1996 Blacks had the highest death rates of any ethnic group for seven of the ten leading causes of death: heart disease, stroke, diabetes, lung cancer, colorectal cancer, breast cancer, pneumonia, and influenza (*Morbidity and Mortality Weekly Review* 2000; Williams 1998). In 1990 the age-adjusted death rate was higher among Blacks than Whites for thirteen of the fifteen leading causes of death. It was much higher (6.7 times) for homicide, 3.1 times higher for HIV/AIDS, 3.1 times higher for perinatal conditions, 3 times higher for kidney diseases, 2.7 times higher for septicemia, and 2.4 times higher for diabetes. Hispanic Americans and Native Americans also suffered high mortality rates, while Asian Americans had favorable indices.

This is a problem of national significance that will become more and more pressing in the coming decades. While ethnic minorities represented 18 percent of the population in 1970, by 1998 they represented 27 percent, and it is expected that by 2050 their proportion will have increased to nearly 50 percent of all persons in the United States. From 1980 to 1990, African Americans, representing 13 percent of U.S. population, increased from 30 million to 33.5 million. An increase of 1.4 percent per year, this is twice the growth rate of Whites. The Black population figure for 1990 is expected to double to 62 million by the year 2030; 84 percent of this will have been a result of natural increase, the remaining 16 percent from immigration. These demographic changes should influence current national health, education, and welfare policies, in self-defense as well as in consideration of fairness, equity, and a concern for national unity (Shinagawa and Lang 1998). Unless significant policy changes occur in health, welfare, and human services, the general quality of life for all Americans will have deteriorated dramatically by the middle of this century. I believe we have the national talent and resources to meet this challenge, but it will require firm planning and sustained efforts: solutions will not automatically be produced by the economic market. Failure to plan and act could seriously jeopardize our world leadership role.

The U.S. Department of Health and Human Services (HHS) has tried to develop initiatives to improve the health status of minority populations. In 1979 these disparities drew attention with the publication of *Healthy People: The Surgeon General's Report on Health Promotion and Disease Prevention.* The then secretary Margaret Hackler established the Office of Minority Health in 1984 to set goals to reduce these disparities. This was followed by Healthy People 2000 and most recently by Healthy People 2010, which was the third statement of ten-year health objectives for all Americans and which in its last formulation aimed at eliminating, not merely reducing racial and ethnic disparities by 2010. In fiscal year 2002, HHS projected expenditure of 5.7 billion of its 468.8 billion budget on minority health programs, including 158 million for the newly created National Institutes of Health (NIH) National Center on Minority Health and Health Disparities, established in November 2000, which absorbed and elevated the mission and goals of the Office of Research on Minority Health, in existence since 1990. (See HHS 2001.)

On October 26, 1998, the most complete progress review thus far was made of Healthy People 2000 objectives for Black Americans (HHS 1998), revealing progress made from 1987 through 1996. The then surgeon general David Satcher and staff made the presentation to a panel of governmental and nongovernmental experts in the field. Reported health status changes were both favorable and unfavorable. For example life expectancy for Black men increased in 1996 for the third consecutive year to a record 66.1 years, seven years less than for other men; Black women born in 1996 could expect to live to age 74, five years less than for other women.

Age-adjusted death rates met the targets set by the Healthy People 2000 projection in the following conditions: all cancers, hepatitis B, lung cancer, and unintentional injury. However, these reductions will not approach parity with the general population. The most encouraging report was that the number of Black women who had breast exams and mammograms will reach parity. Similar good news was seen in reduced percentage of low birth weight babies and in infant mortality, but there was no change in percentage of very low birth weight babies, and none of these infant-related conditions will meet general population parity. Similarly, while the homicide rate for Black men slowly declined in the 1990s, the rate will continue to be several times greater than for all other men. Coronary heart disease deaths steadily declined during the last decade, and the Healthy People 2000 target will be met. Several other indicators were improving but not fast enough to reach target: breast cancer deaths, tuberculosis, early prenatal care, hospitalization for pelvic inflammatory disease, primary and secondary syphilis, pneumococcal and influenza vaccinations. Several other indicators were dramatically worse: HIV/AIDS; asthma hospitalizations and deaths; diabetes-related deaths; maternal mortality, which is five times greater than for White women; end-stage renal disease; and lower extremity amputation. In all candor, it does not appear that significant overall reductions in health disparities are occurring.

An important next question is, are these health disparities due to disparities in health care delivered to Black Americans? In March 2002 the prestigious Institute of Medicine announced their 562-page report, in which the institute reviewed more than one hundred of the best studies and concluded that ethnic minorities who have the same income, insurance coverage, and medical conditions as Whites receive decidedly poorer care. Among the five major findings were their first: "Finding 1-1: Racial and ethnic disparities in health care exist and, because they are associated with worse outcomes in many cases, are unacceptable" and their second (Finding 2-1), "Racial and ethnic disparities in health care occur in the context of broader historic and contemporary social and economic inequality, and evidence of persistent racial and ethnic discrimination in many sectors of American life" (Smedley, Stith, and Nelson 2002, 17).

Among their recommendations, the foremost and general one relates to increasing the awareness of these disparities among the general public and key stakeholders, especially physicians and providers of care, and to "increas[ing] the proportion of underrepresented U.S. racial and ethnic minorities among health professionals" (Smedley, Stith, and Nelson 2002, 18). In response to a growing awareness of the need for fundamental change in the American health care system, an earlier report of the Institute of Medicine's committee on the quality of health care (Committee on Quality of Health Care in America 2001) listed six aims over the next ten years: to make the health care system more safe, effective, patient-centered, timely, efficient, and equitable. Equity was conceived as being addressed at the levels of both population group equity and the individual patient: "the quality of care should not differ because of such characteris-

tics as gender, race, age, ethnicity, income, education, disability, sexual orientation, or location of residence (Committee on Quality of Health Care
in America 2001, 5–6, 53). Important documentation of these current
needs was presented by the Commonwealth Fund's national survey, which
showed that 30 percent of African Americans notably by age fifty but
across all age groups are living with higher rates of chronic illness but are
more likely to have been uninsured in the past year, compared with 46
percent of Hispanics, 20 percent of Whites, and 21 percent of Asians.
Blacks also are less likely than Whites to have a regular doctor (the survey
indicated that 28 percent of Blacks, as compared with 19 percent of
Whites, do not have a regular doctor), and a greater percentage of Blacks
(23 percent) than Whites (16 percent) report problems communicating
with their doctor. Equal percentages of Blacks and Whites (16 percent in
each case) feel that their doctor has treated them with disrespect (Collins,
Tenny, and Hughes 2002).

Further corroboration of specific problems of physicians relating to
Black patients was found in the large 2001 national survey of 2,608 physicians and of 3,884 members of the general public (Kaiser Family Foundation 2002). Only a minority of physicians believe that the health care system very often treats people unfairly based on the patients' monetary
resources, (47 percent), fluency in English (43 percent), educational status
(39 percent), racial or ethnic background (29 percent), sexual orientation
(23 percent), having a disability (23 percent), or gender (15 percent). However, when responses were tabulated on the basis of the racial or ethnic
background of the physician great differences of perception were revealed.
To the question, do you perceive that members of minority groups receive
unfair treatment "rarely or never" the following percentages of physicians
responded affirmatively: White (75 percent), Asian (65 percent), Latino
(47 percent), African American (22 percent). Similar questions about discrimination occurring "rarely or never" on the basis of other variables received similar percentages of affirmative responses: educational status—
White (62 percent), Asian (64 percent), Latino (49 percent), African
American (27 percent); fluency in English—White (57 percent), Asian (55
percent), Latino (37 percent), African American (26 percent); monetary
resources—White (57 percent), Asian (55 percent), Latino (37 percent),
African American (26 percent). Female physicians were also more likely
than male physicians to say there was unfair treatment based on race or
ethnicity of the patient: female (33 percent), male (10 percent). Female
physicians also perceived more unfairness based on the patient's English
fluency—a 24 percent difference; on whether the patient is male or

female—a 23 percent difference; and because the patient was disabled—
an 18 percent point difference. Even the general population is more likely
than physicians to see unfairness based on the patient's monetary resources—a 24 percent gap; ethnic background—an 18 percent gap; disability—a 17 percent gap; English fluency—a 15 percent gap; sexual orientation—a 13 percent gap; gender—a 12 percent gap; and education—a
9 percent gap. With these findings alone we can see how far apart we can
be even as to the perception of a problem requiring solution. But we can
see also how fortunate it is for the American people that the profession of
medicine is becoming more inclusive of persons from diverse backgrounds. Physicians, like other people, tend to see what they look for, including problems and solutions, all of which means that we need many
sets of eyes and ears and minds working toward building a better health
care system.

There can be no denial that we are in the process of reinventing the
American health care system. In the 1980s, a new set of challenges arose.
Conventional fee-for-service medicine was failing to contain the runaway
escalation of health care costs. Neither doctors nor patients nor hospitals
could control their demands for increasingly costly new forms of care de-
riving from new technological discoveries. Since third-party payers, insurance companies, and the government paid the bills, there was no immediate restraint on medical providers. Both Republican and Democratic
administrations failed to contain these costs. Managed care organizations
(MCOs) arose on the scene, competing with each other to provide all
medical care to a defined group of enrolled persons, promising to hold
down costs by controlling physician and hospital decisions through requirements for prior approval. This increased commercialization of medical care has completely transformed the field (Fuchs 1998, 9–29; Ludmerer 1999, 349–70). Quite aside from the fact that 44 million people have
no health care coverage and are therefore left out of the system, MCOs are
tempted to provide the least possible amount of care and not to enroll
high-risk populations who would reduce profit margins. Physicians are, in
fact, in some cases rewarded in their paychecks for providing *less* treatment
to patients. It comes as no surprise, then, that managed care increases the
vulnerability of poorer and minority patients. Because poverty and ethnicity are closely intertwined and are known to be associated with adverse
health outcomes, quality performance measures could be used to guide
corrections of inadequate medical care.

Many of these problems can be solved by a resolute use of existing resources as well as new system changes (Fiscella et al. 2000). Fiscella et al.

propose five principles that could address these disparate outcomes under existing laws, rules, and regulations of accrediting and reimbursement agencies.

1. The problem must be addressed and services allocated by considering not just medical diagnosis but also the poverty or ethnicity of the patient.
2. A new mandate from the president, Health and Human Services, organized medicine and public health, and general public leadership should include requests for new funds to allow the collection of class-based and ethnic-based information by managed care organizations as well as other providers who would not otherwise develop a new and uniform data collection procedure.
3. Existing quality performance measures should explicitly address poverty and ethnic group membership.
4. Population and regional benchmarks for standards of performance should monitor whether vulnerable groups are being enrolled or disenrolled, as well as being provided with adequate care as determined by preestablished standards.
5. Reimbursement rates should be adjusted to compensate plans for the quality of care provided to these vulnerable groups, and to disaccredit providers who are unwilling to be held accountable (Fiscella et al. 2000, 2581).

These measures would, of course, require political leadership, and taking into account concerns for privacy could firmly link the national objective of eliminating racial/ethnic health disparity to continuing quality improvement methodology (Fiscella et al. 2000, 2581–82). (Some patients might object to identifying themselves by race or ethnicity, and some hospitals might resist receiving a report card showing their treatment outcomes along ethnic and income class lines. Fiscella et al. state "Public input to discussions regarding the tension between the right to privacy and equity in health care are essential" [2582].) David Barton Smith (1999, 312–36) summarizes indicators by means of which communities, health plans, and health care organizations could be monitored on their achievements in reducing racial health disparities.

In 1900 life expectancy at birth was forty-eight years for Whites and thirty-three years for Blacks. Over the next century the quality of life for both groups improved dramatically, so that by 1990 life expectancy was seventy-six years for Whites and sixty-nine years for Blacks. Moreover, the gap between the two groups was reduced from 14.6 to 7.0 years. Yet Blacks are in the position now that Whites were forty years earlier. Throughout the last century Black family income has remained in the range of 50 to

60 percent that of Whites, while the disparity in family wealth is even more severe. The net household wealth for Whites is ten times greater than that of Blacks: among families in the lowest quintile of income the median net worth of Black households is *one dollar*. (The comparable figure for Whites is over ten thousand dollars.) Differential in home ownership is the primary reason for this difference.

Blacks pay a hidden tax because of color, as was demonstrated in a 1990 study of gender and racial/ethnic discrimination in purchase price of new cars. Black and White male and female test buyers found these dramatic differences: White men were offered the best price, White women paid a 40 percent markup, Black men a 200 percent markup, and Black women a massive 300 percent markup. Likewise, most goods and services are priced higher in the Black inner city than in the more affluent suburbs (Ayres 1991).

During the 1990–91 economic downturn Black Americans had a net job loss of 59,500 jobs, while Whites gained 71,000, Asians 55,100, and Latinos 60,000 (Williams 1998, 309). Last hired and first fired is still the signature of the color caste system. Unemployed men cannot marry and provide for their children or inspire them to go to college. Chronically high unemployment rates are an example of institutionalized racism, but a man who loses his job during a recession cannot successfully bring a lawsuit against his employer. Seniority rights automatically strike down those who are last hired. These social realities have relevance to the fact that in 1980 Blacks sustained 59,000 preventable deaths, roughly twice as many as Whites (William 1998). Matters worsened by 1991, when Blacks suffered 66,000 preventable deaths (302). If these matters were more widely known, and this knowledge wisely used to guide the nation's health and socioeconomic policy, we would create a stronger, healthier, and higher quality of life for all Americans. In the broadest context this would be affirmative action in medicine.

The book is organized into three parts. Part I discusses the purpose and history of affirmative action in U.S. medical schools and the history of civil rights in health care, and provides a case study of Cornell University medical college. Part II presents data on approximately 2,000 minority and nonminority medical students throughout the country who graduated during the five year period from 1973 to 1977, analyzing the hospitals they selected for post graduate training, the geographic and specialty distribution of these programs and affirmative action in graduate medical education. In part III this cohort was followed up 30 years later, utilizing data showing their practice location and specialty distribution in 1994 and 1995. A final chapter draws from the previous chapters, and my own experiences, to offer my opinions on the future of affirmative action in medical education.

PART I

1. Affirmative Action

IN U.S. MEDICAL SCHOOLS

AFFIRMATIVE ACTION is a deliberate race-conscious recruitment goal designed to equalize access within a set time frame to the high-status jobs and professions such as medicine, from which Blacks have been unfairly excluded for many generations. The concept is based on the premise that relief from illegal racial discrimination is not enough to remove the burden of second-class citizenship from Blacks and other underrepresented minority groups in the United States. In the case of Blacks, for example, slavery and later the imposition of compulsory racial segregation and inferior public and private services were protected government actions. Affirmative action, aided by the same government, is therefore both justified and required to fulfill the objective of equal access. Meaningful equality can only be measured by equal results; otherwise equal opportunity lacks essential meaning, since the social system given a tendency to repeat past history will automatically militate against the equal treatment of minority groups.[1]

Therefore, if the student body, faculty, and administration in a professional school reveal a pattern of minority underrepresentation, despite the presence of a qualified minority applicant pool from which more selections could have been made, it can be assumed that they are being denied essentially equal access or opportunity. Such an institution would be ineligible to receive federal funds and would be required by federal law to draw up a corrective affirmative action plan. This plan is updated annually and establishes the means and methods for recruiting a more equal proportion of minority individuals into the higher levels of the institution's status hierarchy. Affirmative action efforts are subject to federal review, which determines whether they have been carried out in good faith, are adequately documented, and have satisfactory results. The regulations cannot be satisfied by merely going through the motions and completing a set of forms. Affirmative action plans are not explicitly required for admission of students to graduate or professional schools, although they are

13

required for hiring faculty and staff and probably also postgraduate trainees, who are both students and employees simultaneously. Proponents of affirmative action argue that student admissions are covered implicitly, inasmuch as entry to professional school is an absolute determinant of one's future access to professional employment as a faculty member, researcher, or medical practitioner (Institute for the Study of Educational Policy 1976; Fleming, Gill, and Swinton, 1978; C. J. Smith 1978).

The U.S. Commission on Civil Rights concurs that the same constitutional guarantees that protect equal minority access to employment also cover access to admission to professional schools because they are the gateway to professional employment (U.S. Commission on Civil Rights 1977, 1978). All preadmission tests must have a valid and demonstrable relationship to the applicant's ability to perform defined job-related tasks and cannot be used as a device to discriminate racially. The Carnegie Council on Policy Studies in Higher Education (1977, 2–18) concluded that the public policy gains from affirmative race-conscious admissions programs could be achieved without sacrificing essential academic standards, as long as only qualified minority applicants are accepted. This chapter focuses on medical school admissions past and present, and how admissions practices particularly have been changed by affirmative action policy since 1968. The study here provides a close-up view of the impact of affirmative action on the field of medicine.

Holzer and Neumark (2000) have given the most up-to-date critical review and assessment of affirmative action not only in college admissions but also in employment and job promotion and in awarding government contracts. Careful research, in their opinion, does not fully support those who either favor or oppose this hotly contested policy (483). The weight of evidence, however, "supports the view that the significant gains made in recent decades by minorities and women have been achieved with relatively small efficiency consequences" (559). Moreover, they conclude that past as well as current discrimination against these groups might well be worsened by a color-blind approach such as use of income level as a selection factor since low-income Whites outnumber Blacks by a wide margin (561).

HOW AFFIRMATIVE ACTION WORKS

The following scenarios depict the kinds of concrete situations that regularly confront medical school admissions committees.

Scenario 1. Suppose it is late in the admissions season. Two applicants are being considered at a medical school, but there is room to admit only one. One applicant, who is Black, is thought by a majority of the mem-

~~bers of the admissions committee to be unqualified, and the rest consider~~
him to be a borderline candidate at best. The other applicant is White and
is considered by all members of the committee to be far from outstanding
but definitely qualified.

In this case the White applicant would be accepted even if no Black students were enrolled at that medical school. Affirmative action does not require that unqualified minority applicants be admitted, and very likely the
Black applicant would not be able to perform satisfactorily as a medical
student nor subsequently as a competent member of the profession. It
would not be good academic or public policy to favor his admission.

Some individuals persist in their beliefs that affirmative action means
that unqualified applicants have to be accepted. It has even been suggested
that some schools have knowingly admitted unqualified applicants in
order to discredit minority admissions programs and give them short lives
in their institutions. In 1969 one medical school in the New York area admitted 14 minority students, of whom only four performed satisfactorily
in the first year; in the same year another school admitted eight, of whom
five repeated the year and required extensive tutoring, creating serious faculty resistance (Curtis 1971, 123–24). Ten years later both schools had admitted only four to six students in subsequent years judging from enrollment data on minority students enrolled and graduating (AAMC
1982–83). Frequently, however, opinions differ on which of two applicants
is more qualified, as well as on the operational definitions of such terms as
qualified, borderline qualified, unqualified, or *highly qualified.* These judgments are influenced by the presence or absence of racial bias, as well as a
host of other considerations. The complexity of this issue will be more
fully explored later in this chapter, and more will be revealed about the
way admissions committees struggle with these matters.

Scenario 2. Again two applicants are being considered, and only one
can be offered acceptance. In the opinion of almost all members of the
admissions committee one applicant, who is Black, is more highly qualified than the other applicant, who is White. The Black applicant seems
best on the basis of grades and scores, letters of recommendation, admissions interview, extracurricular and community activities, and other indications of strong motivation and the likelihood that she will contribute
to the medical profession as a leader. In this case the Black applicant
should be accepted, and most persons correctly would not consider this
to be an example of affirmative action. This Black applicant should be accepted even if Blacks are not underrepresented at that medical school. Affirmative action is intended to provide a minimally acceptable proportion

of qualified members of minority populations; it establishes a floor, not a ceiling, to assure a minimally acceptable inclusion of members of an excluded group, not the exclusion of any group members after these equitable conditions are met.

Scenario 3. In this situation both the Black and the White applicant are qualified, although neither is exceptional as far as can be determined. This situation occurs far more commonly than either of the two preceding scenarios.

If only one candidate can be offered a place, it is in such an instance that the Black applicant should be accepted, provided that Blacks are significantly underrepresented in the student body of that medical school. This is affirmative action, when qualified members of underrepresented minority groups are admitted until there is a minimally equitable level of representation from the underrepresented group. Swain (2000) states that survey questions can be phrased in such a way, within various contexts, as to obtain contradictory findings on the controversial issue of affirmative action. She states, however, that in a scenario in which both a Black and a White applicant are equally qualified and only one can be accepted, 78 percent of Whites and 72 percent of Blacks believe that race should not be a factor in the admission decision. Some other basis should be found, such as adverse life circumstance versus a background of family comfort and privilege, to determine the admission decision.

The minority population and the size of the applicant pool at local, state, and national levels are useful in determining minimally acceptable and fair levels of representation. The rationale for such action rests not only on the laudable purpose of equalizing the civil and legal rights of all Americans, but also on the grounds that an ethnically diverse student body will, by its very composition, obtain a sounder medical education and as physicians be more responsive to the medical needs of the diverse American public.

WHY AFFIRMATIVE ACTION WAS NECESSARY

Medical education was generally not available to Blacks until 1868, when Howard University Medical School in Washington, D.C., opened its doors. Meharry Medical College in Nashville began operating in 1876. For all practical purposes, these two schools were set aside for Blacks, at a time when all the other medical schools did not accept, or admitted only token numbers of, Blacks (Johnson 1967; Curtis 1971, 34).

The founding of Howard University in 1866 is an example of affirmative action in the period immediately following the Civil War. The

NAACP Legal Defense Fund's amicus brief in the case of the *Regents of the University of California v. Bakke* pointed out that Congress, in framing the Fourteenth Amendment, demonstrated a belief that race-specific remedies are both necessary and permissible and adopted a series of measures that established special educational and medical programs solely for Blacks (NAACP 1976, 12–48). Indeed the Freedman's Bureau Act of 1866, under whose authority Howard and a number of other well-known Black colleges in the South were founded, was enacted over two vetoes by President Andrew Johnson, who opposed special aid for Blacks. A major purpose of the Fourteenth Amendment and its equal protection clause was to assure the constitutionality of the Freedman's Bureau Act. In an era when public education was open to only a few privileged Whites, it is not surprising that many Americans were opposed even to segregated elementary or high schools for Blacks, not to mention Black colleges or professional schools.

Blacks were for the most part excluded from the tremendously increased higher education opportunities that opened up for other Americans during the rapid and extreme expansion of the college and university system following the Civil War through the end of World War II, including the federally funded land grant colleges for Whites (Drake 1971). Had the segregated Black colleges not existed, as a kind of affirmative action program that was better than nothing, Blacks today would suffer a much more grave educational inequality than they do. Following the 1896 *Plessy v. Ferguson* decision of the Supreme Court, racially "separate but equal" facilities became the pattern in public institutions and accommodations, including schools. It was transparently inevitable that separate and inferior Black schools and colleges would permanently assure the systematic undereducation and subordination of Blacks to Whites. Therefore, Black colleges have served two different purposes, depending on the strength, wisdom, and motivations of their leadership. These colleges can promote an affirmative action mission by educating Blacks who otherwise would not be educated, or they can foster a lower standard of education for Blacks. White leaders more than Black have used these colleges for the latter purpose. Perhaps the best example of this is Meharry Medical College, one of the predominantly Black medical schools, which was founded in 1876. The Southern Regional Education Board consisted of representatives from 15 southern and border states to guide their higher educational policies, this policy for Blacks being "separate but equal." As recently as 1968 a majority of Meharry's first year class was set aside for Black students from those states whose education was partly financed to keep them from attending White medical schools in their states of origin (Cogan 1968, 5, 25–26, 59).

BLACK ENROLLMENT IN MEDICAL SCHOOLS

Table 1 shows Black enrollment in U.S. medical schools from 1938 through 1997. In 1938, Blacks were approximately 10 percent of the population but only 1.6 percent of all enrolled medical students. More than 87 percent of them were matriculated at Howard or Meharry. A decade later Black enrollment had increased to 2.6 percent, and just over 84 percent still were enrolled at one of the two predominantly Black medical schools.

In the late 1930s there began a decade of major legal challenges to the constitutionality of racially segregated education (Kluger 1976, 155–238). The NAACP launched a major attack on the separate and unequal graduate and professional schools of the southern states, at first demanding only equal educational treatment. It was thought to be strategically wise first to win a number of cases on the basis of the demonstrable inequality or absence of postgraduate and professional school facilities provided to Blacks, rather than to tackle the fundamental doctrine enthroned under the *Plessy* case, the pretense that racially separate schooling could be equal.

In 1935, Charles Houston, former dean of Howard University Law School and a graduate of Amherst College and Harvard Law School, and one of his extremely able former students, Thurgood Marshall, brought suit against the University of Maryland to admit Donald Murray, a recent Black graduate of Amherst, to its law school. Murray was accepted in 1938, following three years of litigation.

Another student, Lloyd Gaines, was admitted to the University of Missouri Law School after a legal contest also decided by the Supreme Court in 1938. As commonly was done in those days, Missouri had offered to pay

TABLE 1. Enrollment of Blacks in U.S. Medical Schools, 1938–97

	Year	Total Enrollment	Total Black Enrollment	Percentage in Predominantly White Schools	Percentage of All Enrolled Medical Students
Pre–civil rights	1938	21,302	350	12.9	1.6
	1947	22,739	588	15.8	2.6
Desegregation era	1955	28,639	761	31.0	2.7
	1968	35,833	783	37.3	2.2
Affirmative action	1969	37,690	1,042	52.4	2.8
	1977	60,039	3,587	80.0	6.0
	1997	66,900	5,303	86.6	7.9

Sources: Dietrich C. Reitzes, *Negroes and Medicine,* Harvard University Press, 1958; Charles E. Odegaard, *Minorities in Medicine,* The Josiah Macy, Jr. Foundation, 1977; AAMC enrollment data for 1977; AAMC enrollment data for 1997.

tuition for Gaines to attend a law school in any other state in order to keep the state university all White. When he did not agree, the state offered a defense that there were too few Blacks applying to law school in Missouri to warrant the expense of establishing a law school for Blacks only. Chief Justice Charles Evans Hughes ruled that "the State was bound to furnish . . . within its borders facilities for legal education substantially equal to those which the State there afforded for persons of the White race."

Other admissions suits against law schools in Oklahoma and Texas in 1946 were decided similarly in 1948 and 1950. Even though the Court avoided a ruling on the "separate but equal" doctrine, it had already made it clear that a state could not provide an equal professional education for Blacks by setting up a small pretense of a school, which lacked comparable student-faculty-alumni supportive networks, comparable libraries, or comparable reputations for excellence. Writing for a unanimous Supreme Court on June 5, 1950, Chief Justice Vinson stated that in both Oklahoma and Texas "we cannot find substantial equality in the educational opportunities offered White and Negro law students by the state" (Kluger 1976, 282). A 1942 U.S. Office of Education survey of higher educational opportunity for Blacks in the seventeen southern and border states revealed that segregated schools were mandatory in all of them either by state constitution or statute, that professional and graduate educational offerings were not equal anywhere, and that, for example, in sixteen states a law curriculum was offered for Whites but was available in only two states for Blacks. In 1940 about 80 percent of all Blacks lived in those states; 70 percent still lived there in the 1950s. Medical education was offered to Whites in thirteen of the seventeen states and the District of Columbia, but was offered to Blacks only in the two states where Howard and Meharry were located.

When I was admitted to the University of Michigan in 1943 I was the only Black student in a class originally of 175 and of whom 145 graduated. Probably I was the only Black student that year as a consequence of military service. Already accepted into the Medical School I was drafted and as a result of my test scores was made a member of the Army Specialist Training Corps for Blacks, since the military was at that time segregated. I was slated to study engineering, but because I had already been accepted for the Michigan Medical School, Albion College and the University of Michigan requested that I go to Medical School. On arriving I noticed that each class had two Black students, and in the course of my years there each year they admitted two or three Black students. All enrolled students were members of the Army Specialist Training Corps (ASTP) or the Navy V12 program except for the small number of six or so women in each class.

Men lived in the Victor Vaughn Medical Dormitory for men except for those preferring to live in their White fraternity house. That was the first year Blacks lived in the dormitory for men because dormitories at Michigan then were segregated. When I was in my junior year and the war ended, I completed school as a civilian and was required to rent quarters off campus. During those medical school years I made many friends of different races since all of my earlier schooling had been in racially integrated schools where I was the only or one of only a few Blacks in a class. In my graduating class of 145 I finished twenty-eighth.

LEGAL DESEGREGATION

The Supreme Court's 1954 decision in *Brown v. Board of Education* ended the *Plessy* doctrine of "separate but equal." Chief Justice Earl Warren found that to segregate children racially in public schools in and of itself deprived minority children of an equal education guaranteed them by the equal protection clause of the Fourteenth Amendment. Public schools in the lower levels were inherently unequal simply by virtue of their being racially segregated.

Some of the southern states refused to recognize that *Brown* applied to graduate and professional schools as well as elementary and high schools. North Carolina, Alabama, Tennessee, Georgia, Louisiana, Mississippi, and Florida all brought legal tests of the issue. In *Frazier v. the Board of Trustees of the University of North Carolina* the Supreme Court stood firm in its 1956 decision that the reasoning in *Brown* applied with equal force to colleges: "Indeed it is fair to say that they apply with greater force to students of mature age in the concluding years of their formal education as they are about to engage in the serious business of adult life" (Amicus brief in *California v. Bakke*, National Fund for Minority Engineering Students 1976).

The legal struggle to maintain segregated higher education dwindled in the mid-1960s. However, in 1968, fourteen years after Blacks had won a major constitutional law victory, only twenty-two more Black students were enrolled in the nation's medical schools than were registered when the Supreme Court pronounced the verdict in *Brown*. At this time, though, the entire nation developed a mood of willingness to begin to correct the social injustices long inflicted on Blacks. Reasons for this change included the nonviolent civil rights movement led by Martin Luther King Jr.; the student protest against the Vietnam War and social injustice generally; the urban riots by Blacks, especially following King's assassination; and the development of increasing Black militance (Grimshaw 1969; Ludmerer 1999, 250–53). Between 1968 and 1969, Black enrollment in U.S.

medical schools increased from 783 to 1,042. Even more dramatic for that one-year period was the percentage enrolled in predominantly White schools, an increase from 37.3 percent to 52.4 percent. By 1977, Black enrollment had increased to 3,587, or 6 percent of the total medical school enrollment, with 80 percent of the students enrolled in predominantly White schools. Although this figure did not approach the 11 percent total proportion of Black individuals in the population, it represented a significant improvement over any previous era. Progress continued up to 1997, when Black enrollment was 7.9 percent but still below target.

Wellington and Montero (1978) surveyed the affirmative action programs for minority students in the 112 U.S. medical schools and rated the effectiveness of the various components in their equal education efforts. By far the most significant effort was the modification of traditional admission criteria in order to recruit and admit more minority students. Invariably this was done more successfully when minority group individuals sat on admissions committees. In addition, considerable effort went into providing additional student aid in the form of counseling, tutoring, and financial aid support for minority students. By their own rating, medical schools had been significantly less successful in their recruitment of minority faculty and administrators between 1968 and 1972, and indeed there continued to be very little change in that picture up to 1976 and even until 1996 when the percentage of Black faculty was only 2.6 (AAMC 1998). (Descriptions of the development and course of minority medical school enrollment can be found in Curtis 1971, which covers the years up to 1970; Odegaard 1977, which covers the period from 1966 to 1976; Shea and Fullilove 1985; Watson 1999, 19–43; and Ludmerer 1999, 251–56.)

THE *BAKKE* CONFRONTATION

Arguments for and against affirmative action were presented in the more than sixty legal briefs presented to the Supreme Court in the case of *Regents of the University of California v. Bakke.* The Association of American Medical Colleges (AAMC) submitted a brief supporting the preferential admissions program of the University of California (Davis) Medical College (AAMC 1976). Allan Bakke, an engineer who at age thirty-three decided to apply to medical schools, was turned down for two years by all schools to which he applied. His second application to the University of California (Davis) was thought to be unsuccessful because he made a poor interview impression, and from my experience on an admission committee I would surmise also that his age and his second choice of medicine were factors against him. He claimed that because UC Davis set aside 16 of its 100 places in the entering class for minority students that he had suffered illegal racial discrimination since his grade point average and scores were higher than those of minority students admitted under a quota plan.

The AAMC had an important stake in the outcome of this dispute because in 1968 it had urged all medical schools to voluntarily admit increased numbers of students from geographic areas, economic backgrounds, and ethnic groups that were inadequately represented (AAMC 1968). Specific emphasis on the importance of the race-consciousness in this affirmative action program was further underscored by the 1970 national task force report (AAMC 1970) on ways to expand educational opportunities in medicine for Blacks and other underrepresented minorities (specifically also Hispanics and Native Americans). A specific affirmative action goal was set to raise enrollment from a level of just over 2 percent to 12 percent by 1975. Other medical organizations, including the American Hospital Association, the American Medical Association, and the National Medical Association, had joined the AAMC in endorsing this affirmative action effort. It is worth noting that the NMA was formed in 1895 because the AMA refused to accept Blacks as members. Indeed it was not until 1968 that the AMA prohibited racial bars to membership in all of its state and local branches. In the spirit of the late 1960s, therefore, even the conservative medical establishment supported the need for special programs to bring about more equal medical educational opportunities for Blacks and other excluded minority groups. Although the goal of 12 percent was not attained in 1975, it reached 10 percent by that year. It was disquieting to note that from 1975 on, first-year minority enrollment slumped to 9 percent and then to just under 8 percent by 1978, an indication that affirmative action efforts did not rest on secure ground.

In its *Statement on Affirmative Action* (1977), the U.S. Commission on Civil Rights called attention to some of the shortcomings in the University of California defense of its affirmative action program; their criticism applied with equal force to the legal brief submitted by the AAMC (1976). Medical schools were less than candid about their intended or unintended prior exclusion of minorities, and their case would have been strengthened had they been more forthright in such a statement. Most professional schools, and this was especially the case with the state university system in California, were reluctant to go on record with an acknowledgment of their own previous record of racial discrimination in admission or hiring of minorities. Furthermore, public universities usually are reluctant to cite other public agencies, such as public schools and college systems in their own state that, in effect, deny equal educational opportunity, and thereby equal minority student access to graduate or professional school admission. The professional schools often are not on public record concerning the limitations of admissions tests or grade point averages in forecasting future student or professional success; nor are they on record in stating that an important mission of their school is to provide physicians to serve all of the people in their state (U.S. Commission on Civil Rights 1977).

The defense of affirmative action programs in *Bakke* rested on the following points: (1) the low representation of minorities in professional schools and in the profession, (2) the benefits to students, especially nonminority students, of receiving an education as part of an ethnically diverse student body, (3) the need to train minority professionals to serve as role models and sources of inspiration and hope to aspiring minority youngsters, (4) the need to train increased numbers of minority professionals, who would improve services to the underserved minority communities, (5) the need to improve the ability and willingness of future nonminority physicians to serve more effectively in minority communities, (6) and the need to evaluate more closely personal attributes and life experience of minority applicants to assure that their potential abilities are not underestimated (Brief for Petitioner 1976).

In June 1978 the Supreme Court decided that medical schools could use race as one factor in affirmative action admissions as long as other factors, such as special qualities an individual applicant might bring to his or her class, also were allowed. However, a medical school could not set up an arbitrary quota or reserve seats only for members of any specific racial group. The University of California at Davis was the only public medical school in the nation that operated under a stated quota system and with a separate admissions committee for minority applicants. The university also tacitly confessed that Allan Bakke was more qualified than some minority students who were admitted and that he would have been admitted had there not been a minority quota.

Some civil rights proponents believed that the University of California had deliberately put its worst foot forward and should drop the case, pointing out that a member of its admissions committee had advised Bakke to bring suit. In addition the university did not establish a need for its minority program in pretrial arguments (Dreyfuss and Lawrence 1979; Tollett 1978; Burke 1977). Most regrettable was the fact that the Supreme Court justices were unable to come to a unanimous opinion.

THE MEDICAL SCHOOL ADMISSIONS
PROCESS EXAMINED

DEFINING THE QUALIFIED APPLICANT

Medical schools throughout the country annually face the task of selecting those applicants who will become the most able, willing, and successful medical students and, even more, who will best serve the need for future physicians as practitioners, researchers, teachers, and administrators.
As the AAMC pointed out in their amicus brief in the *Bakke* case, during
the 1960s the competition to get into medical school became increasingly
intense, the number of applicants having approximately tripled while the
number of first-year places only doubled. This doubling occurred in response to increasing public pressure for better health care delivery. The
large increase in the number of applicants was largely a response to reduced opportunity in graduate-level Ph.D. and engineering programs,
and it created an especially difficult political problem. Indeed Bakke's decision to switch fields to medicine, coupled with his age, probably accounted for the fact that over a two-year period he was rejected by a dozen
medical schools. Affirmative action admissions programs for qualified minority students would have been difficult in normal times, given the fact
that their traditional educational racial handicap left them with test scores
attained two decades or so earlier by Whites.

Table 2 shows that the number of applicants increased from 1967 to 1975,
as did the percentage of those accepted who had A averages. Subtest scores
on the Medical College Admissions Test (MCAT) also increased. The average admission test scores for Black students accepted into medical schools
during the period from 1967 to 1975 were a hundred points lower than those
of nonminority students. As the AAMC brief points out, although the
scores of Blacks were the same as those earned by Whites twenty years ear-

TABLE 2. **Mean MCAT Scores and GPAs for Accepted Medical Students,
1967–75**

Year	Number of Applicants	Percentage Accepted	Mean Subtest Scores		GPA	
			Quantitative	Science	A (3.6–4.0)	B (2.6–3.5)
1967	18,724	51.8	596	565	14.1%	76.8%
1972	36,135	38.1	614	575	28.9%	60.1%
1975	42,303	36.3	620	615	44.2%	47.4%

Source: Carnegie Council on Policy Studies in Higher Education 1977, appendixes D-1, D-8.

lier and were high enough to reflect adequate academic qualification and merit, this fact was generally not understood by the public.

Since Blacks and other minority students have to perform the same academic work as all other medical students, it would be reasonable to expect that minority students would encounter more than an average amount of academic difficulty. Indeed retention rates for Blacks at the end of their first year were only 95 percent and 91 percent in 1970 and 1971, compared with 98 percent and 97 percent for White students. More Black students were dropped, but the demand for maintenance of standards in the face of unequal preparation would necessarily have led to that result. I believe this could also be taken as a sign of reasonable academic responsibility and risk taking, that medical school faculties were accepting the difficult social challenge of democratizing the future physician manpower of the nation.

On the other hand, critics of affirmative action programs have persistently maintained that MCAT scores and grade point averages are fixed measures of meritorious achievement and qualification, without consideration of the different learning backgrounds in which these scores and grades are obtained. The AAMC countered these arguments (Petersdorf et al. 1990, esp. 665–66) by pointing out that although grades and admissions test scores have some predictive power for the first two years of basic science medical school course work, this power is limited for all students for the last two years of clinical work or for future medical career success. For these reasons medical school admissions committees always place considerable emphasis on letters of recommendation from the premedical advisors and other faculty members, review of the applicant's autobiographical statement, even though others may have helped to write it, and breadth of extracurricular and community interests. Of even greater importance are the interviews with members of the admissions committee to determine an applicant's maturity, stability, motivation for a career in medicine, depth of interest in the field, and ability to relate to and communicate with others. An estimate of these subjective factors before the interview plays a large role in deciding which applicants will be invited for interviews.

DECISIONS ON MAKING UP THE CLASS

The easy decisions regarding admissions involve only a fraction of those who are interviewed. Most medical schools usually are left with several hundred or several thousand of qualified but not exceptional applicants, while places can be offered only to about a hundred. Why should an applicant's race be a relevant factor favoring him or her over another applicant with essentially similar qualifications?

When he was president of the Ford Foundation, McGeorge Bundy (1977) pointed out that in 1975–76, there were just under 35,000 White applicants to medical schools, of whom 22,000 were not accepted. In that same year, the total number of minority applicants accepted and enrolled was 1,400. If not a single minority applicant had been accepted, there would still have been more than 20,600 disappointed White applicants. In other words, the question becomes one of whether or not the nation stands to gain more by reducing White applicant disappointment by a mere 7 percent, or by making a major and sizable improvement in broadening the medical representation of minority groups (almost a sevenfold numerical increase over traditional minority enrollment levels).

Most people who have had no experience with admissions decisions are unaware that a mixture of aims must be satisfied in the selection of an entering class. From experience on a medical school admissions committee in the 1970s, I only gradually came to appreciate the complexity of the admissions process. Even if it were possible to assess all of an applicant's cognitive and noncognitive assets and liabilities, it is impossible to judge how that applicant would have looked coming from a different background, or will look four years later in a new environment. Admissions committees do not have a high batting average in selecting students who, four years later, will prove to have been as outstanding, excellent, or extraordinary as was predicted in the admissions year. About 10 percent of a class is usually predicted to be in the highest category of excellence. At best only a third of them perform up to expectation in their subsequent school work, and a substantial proportion of those predicted to be average have been found to be very much better or worse than anticipated.

While I was on the medical school admissions committee in the 1970s, the Cornell University Medical College committee interviewed approximately 1,000 of its 6,000 or so applicants; of those, perhaps 800 were considered acceptable. Acceptable applicants were then rated into one of five degrees of acceptability. Usually only people in the two top categories were offered admission. In order to constitute a class of 101 students, about 180 acceptances were offered. But two minority students had to be accepted to obtain one enrollment, since the "best" minority students are fewer in number. Students who were accepted at Cornell ordinarily had been accepted by most of the other medical schools to which they applied. Medical schools therefore compete for the "best" applicants, making admissions decisions a two-way process involving both the applicant and the school.

Some factors have little direct relationship to personal attributes of an applicant but great bearing on whether he or she will be chosen as a member of that class. These include whether or not the applicant is a resident of the state in which the school is located, since all medical schools in most states suffer financial penalties of reduced state support unless they enroll a majority of state residents. This was surely the case in New York. The Health Professions Educational Assistance Act of 1976 and subsequent amendments denied federal funding to medical schools unless (1) 50 percent or more of its graduates selected primary care residency training programs, (2) capitation awards were made to students who agreed in writing that they would practice for a year in an underserved area, and (3) that a quota of Americans who completed the first two years of their medical education abroad would be admitted as third-year students to American Medical schools (Ludmerer 1999, chap. 19).

Attention also was given to whether or not the first-year applicant came from one's own undergraduate college campus. Ordinarily about one-sixth to one-fifth of the entering class came from Cornell, although the entire class usually could have been filled with acceptable Cornell graduates. Special preference also was given to children of faculty members, and lesser but some attention was given to children of alumni and the spouses of enrolled students.

In order to obtain geographic and social diversity, an effort was made to admit a few students from schools in different parts of the country, and to admit some students from public as well as from private schools, although a definite preference went to applicants from prestigious institutions, whether public or private. Admissions committees have enough flexibility to bend their admissions to serve a number of purposes, as long as the accepted student does not carry too great a percentage of academic risk. However, this is only the beginning.

Suppose it had been observed that a significant proportion (4 percent to 6 percent) of students traditionally had come from prestige university A, but for some reason very few students from that school had applied in a given year. Further, of those who did apply fewer elected to enroll. An informal investigation usually would reveal that another medical school, one or several of Cornell's peers, had developed a new and special competitive advantage over Cornell. An effort would then be mounted to restore Cornell's former position. This may have involved accepting more than the usual number of students from that school, actively recruiting more applicants, possibly even accepting a few students who previously would not have been accepted, and attempting especially to counteract any negative rumor that might have been circulated concerning Cornell.

Conversely, if too many students from a particular university were found to be highly acceptable, some might not be offered places simply because they would represent an unusually large proportion of the whole CUMC class. In other words, the decision to admit a student from a particular college or university is inextricably involved in the status struggle between medical schools, each school being constrained to maintain or improve its competitive position and prestige image within the system. Premed advisors at the various colleges are also compelled to build up the image of their schools, and for this reason they influence the numbers of applicants who apply to this or that medical school, so that their applicants do not cancel out each other's chances of being accepted.

Medical schools must compete to attract the most able applicants from the high-prestige colleges and universities, and such applicants never lack schools they can choose or reject. In fact by listening to the many able applicants to a medical school each year, one learns how the outside world is perceiving one's school and is compelled to ponder problems that require correction. It is healthy for a medical school, like any other institution in a responsible society, to hear the contribution it is making to the healthy development and growth of that society, and to be held accountable for its efforts. Ultimately neither strong students, faculty, nor administration will choose to be part of a school that does not merit their continuing respect. Thus, as I described in my previous book (Curtis 1971), a group of medical students and faculty at Cornell in 1968 were concerned that their school was not following the lead of schools like Harvard, Stanford, or Columbia in admitting qualified minority students. They pressured the entire faculty and administration to make a formal commitment to enroll a class with 10 percent Black students and to recruit qualified Black faculty leadership to develop an effective program. After I was appointed to the faculty and dean's staff, I was prominently involved in interviewing both minority and nonminority applicants in order to send the message that Cornell wanted to change its image as an all-White medical school. One cannot overestimate the influence of peer institutional pressure in exacting socially acceptable and responsible behavior from medical schools.

CHANGES IN COMPOSITION OF THE MEDICAL STUDENT BODY OVER THE YEARS

Between 1968 and 1978 the number of medical schools in the United States increased from 99 to 124 (35.3 percent increase), and the total number of enrolled students rose from 35,833 to 62,242 (67.6 percent increase). During the same period, there was a major shift in gender of enrolled students, with females increasing from 8.8 percent to 24.3 percent. Enrollment of underrepresented minorities increased from 2.4 percent to 7.9 percent. The corresponding increase for U.S. Blacks was from 2.2 percent to 5.7 percent. The steady increase in enrollment of women, which, except during World War II, had been restricted to approximately 5 to 6 percent, was a direct response to affirmative action efforts, which were strengthened by the 1972 education amendments prohibiting discrimination against women in admissions or in other aspects of student programs and services. This achievement was accomplished with very little in the way of public notice, acclaim, or controversy.

In the late 1960s many schools automatically returned applications submitted by persons over the age of twenty-six, but today nearly all schools annually enroll students in their thirties and older, some of whom are married and have children. Those older students bring with them greater maturity and important experiences from other careers. Similarly there are more physically handicapped persons, again in response to affirmative action efforts either mandated or voluntarily undertaken.

FOREIGN MEDICAL SCHOOLS

The absolute number of applicants to U.S. medical schools declined 15 percent from its peak in 1974–75 to 1979–80, and first-year places expanded by 13.7 percent in the same period. However, there still were 19,127 unsuccessful applicants to U.S. medical schools for the 1979–80 year ("Annual Report" 1980). Those 19,000 rejected applicants exceeded the total of all applicants to U.S. schools in most years prior to 1968, an expression of the tremendous upsurge of the desire of young Americans to become physicians during the 1970s.

In 1980 it was estimated that as many as 11,000 or more U.S. students might be studying medicine abroad, most of them enrolled in half a dozen proprietary schools located in Mexico or the Caribbean. The political influence of the parents of those students, a large fraction of whom were New Yorkers, was believed to be responsible for an unprecedented action by the New York State Board of Regents, which proposed setting up guidelines by means of which the state could approve these foreign schools, whose students would then be eligible to transfer into the third-year classes of medical schools located in New York. This proposed action was at first not supported by the AAMC or the AMA ("New York's Policy" 1980), which jointly operate the medical school accreditation agency, the Liaison Committee on Medical Education. Despite opposition, the medical schools in New York state began admitting these students to their third-year classes—after the AAMC gave official support to this program in 1970 (Ludmerer 1999, 272–75). In the case of Cornell, ten new students from these foreign medical schools were admitted to the third-year class after 1976.

HOW MANY PHYSICIANS DO WE NEED?

By 1980 a consensus had developed that the nation soon would experience a physician surplus. We were graduating students from U.S. medical schools at a rate that had doubled from 1960 to 1980 to almost sixteen thousand graduates a year. By 1985 an estimated total of eleven thousand U.S. citizens were studying medicine abroad, often in substandard medical schools, and there were an equal number of foreign medical school graduates in our residency training programs. It was estimated by an expert panel, the Graduate Medical Education National Advisory Committee (GMENAC), that by 1996 we would have an excess of seventy thousand physicians over the "need." Furthermore, the surplus might be greater still if we made better use of physician's assistants, nurse-practitioners, and other paraprofessional workers. The problem of physician supply was not one of a low absolute number of physicians but rather that many geographical areas, such as rural counties and inner city ghetto neighborhoods, had relatively few doctors and that American physicians were overspecialized in surgical and medical subspecialties with too few giving primary and basic general medical care. GMENAC suggested that U.S. medical school enrollment could be reduced by 17 percent relative to the 1980–81 entering class and that in the future restrictions should be placed on the entry of U.S. citizens and foreign nationals from medical schools abroad. There was a reaffirmed need to improve the diversity of medical school student bodies with regard to "socioeconomic status, sex, and race by providing loans and scholarships to achieve these goals and by emphasizing as role models, women and under-represented minority faculty members." Medical schools did not reduce their admissions, maintaining annual enrollments at approximately sixteen thousand up to the present time. (A summary of the six-volume GMENAC report, with commentary, appeared in the *Chronicle of Higher Education,* October 6, 1980. See HHS 1980 for information on the complete report.)

A comparison of the production of premedical students in the states of New York and California underscores important similarities and differences in their production of premedical students. In 1970 California had the largest population of any state, with about 20 million, or 9.8 percent of the resident civilian population; New York was second, with approximately 18 million, or 9.0 percent. Looking at all applicants to U.S. medical schools in 1975–76, New York was in first place and provided 12.3 percent of all applicants, who generated 22.1 percent of first-year places. Medical schools located in New York enrolled 10.6 percent of all first-year U.S. medical students that year (Gordon and Johnson 1977). However, New Yorkers also were first in percentage of rejected applicants, contributing 12.2 percent of all unsuccessful applicants. In that sense New York was simultaneously the biggest winner and the biggest loser, by the sheer weight of its proportion of the applicant pool.

California ranked second in each of the categories mentioned above: with 9.6 percent of all applicants, who generated 14.5 percent of all applications, and received 8.0 percent of all enrollments, and 10.5 percent of all unsuccessful applicants. Medical schools in California enrolled only 6.4 percent of all first-year U.S. medical students, demonstrating a smaller contribution compared to New York. Both states, however, exported more first year students to other states than they accommodated in total enrollment capacity. Both states also demonstrate the tremendous desire to become a premedical student, and how difficult it will be to control these aspirations.

CONTROLLING POSTGRADUATE TRAINING AND PRACTICE LOCATION

Thoughtful observers like Alexander Leaf (1978) have pointed out that our maldistribution of medical manpower is unlikely to be improved until physicians give up some of their highly valued independence and self-determination. "We must choose whether medicine is to be a privileged franchise to be practiced for personal advantages or whether our role will be to provide for a public need." Meanwhile there would be continuing governmental efforts to influence physician behavior by changing the method of financial support, education, and training, and changing regulatory and reimbursement formulas for individual and institutional health care providers. Completely free choice of behavior by physicians created problems even for states that were apparently well supplied.

Of the 323,200 active physicians in the United States in 1970, New York contained the highest percentage, 13.3 compared to 12.0 for California, which was second. Both states exceeded the national average of 154 physicians per 100,000 population, New York with 263 and California with 194. Our national physician manpower consisted of 81.0 percent who were educated in the United States, 1.9 percent who were educated in Canadian schools, which are accredited similarly, and 17.1 percent who are educated in foreign schools many of which are operated on very different standards. New York accommodated 27.9 percent of all foreign medical graduates (FMGs); attracted 10.3 percent of U.S. graduates and 17.2 percent of Canadian graduates. California relied only on 5.2 percent of the nation's FMGs; contained 13.9 percent of U.S. and 18.2 percent of Canadian medical school graduates.

As early as 1953, New York state repealed its educational requirements for internships in order to fill positions especially in underserved areas (Maynard 1978, 193–99). Not until 1960 did the Educational Committee for Foreign Medical Graduates require passing its certifying exam as a precondition for serving on any hospital house staff in the country. As soon as immigration restrictions were loosened, many FMGs entered residency training programs in New York state and subsequently became medical staff members at a number of hospitals located in minority group and low-income areas. Because they were willing to accept employment at salary levels unacceptable to U.S. graduates, many also began to fill postgraduate and staff positions in the state psychiatric hospitals and institutions for the developmentally disabled.

In 1974, New York offered 9,549 residency training positions, a number amounting to 16.7 percent of all residency positions offered in the United States. While 96 percent of these were filled, only 49 percent were taken by U.S. and Canadian graduates. That same year California offered only 5,593 residency positions, and filled 93 percent. However, 95 percent of the California residents were U.S. or Canadian graduates and only 5 percent were FMGs ("Medical Education in the United States" 1976). In other words, New York and California succeed equally in attracting absolute numbers of U.S. medical school graduates. During the years when immigration restrictions on FMGs were loosened, New York became heavily dependent on these physicians in a pattern unlike that of any other state.

CONTROLLING THE CONTINUUM OF PHYSICIAN MANPOWER PRODUCTION

Realigning the system in a state requires attention to the pool of premedical students, undergraduate medical students, postgraduate trainees in needed fields, and financial and other incentives to encourage physicians to locate in certain areas. Merely establishing a new medical school in an area that is no longer attractive to practicing physicians is not a solution to a shortage. For example, the State University of New York (Downstate Medical Center) was started when the state took over the former Long Island College of Medicine in 1950. According to one of the loudly stated political arguments, that medical school, located in Brooklyn, was set up to train physicians who would remain in the New York metropolitan area. The number of practicing physicians in Brooklyn had fallen from 6,000 in 1960 to 3,600 by 1975, although the population remained at about 2.8 million. There had been a major demographic shift in population, with many middle-income Whites moving to the suburbs and being replaced by low-income Blacks and Puerto Ricans (Fernandes and Imperato 1980).

In a 1981 poll of second-year medical students at SUNY Downstate, Fernandes and Imperato found that only 2.5 percent planned to do their postgraduate training in Brooklyn, and only 3.3 percent were planning to practice there. The authors attributed the students' negative responses and reactions to the unattractive surroundings and quality of life of the inner city neighborhood in which the medical school is located. While this is undoubtedly correct, it is important to note that only 6 (2.7 percent) of the 223 students were minority group members (5 Blacks and 1 Puerto Rican). Large nationwide studies and AAMC annual surveys of graduating students show that a large proportion of minority students plan to pursue future training in inner city hospitals like Kings County, are doing so currently, and plan to practice in the inner city (DHEW 1978b; Petersdorf et al. 1990).

This is an important phenomenon, and it demands further elaboration. In chapter 7 I present data that illustrate the degree to which physicians from underrepresented minority groups who graduated from medical schools in the five-year period from 1969 to 1974, and who were in practice in the 1990s, were providing extensive medical care to members of their minority group in comparison to nonminority peers who finished medical school in the same time period. We found that not only do minority group physicians establish practices where their subpopulations live but that White physicians tend to practice in the more middle income areas where they grew up and reside. For minority group physicians the income of their families of origin did not predict future practice locations.

Because our nation is still racially segregated, and particularly since we have experienced increasingly segregated Black neighborhoods both in cities and suburbs within the past thirty years, members of minority groups will have more immediate access to physicians who belong to their group. Managed care companies state that the preferred doctor-to-patient ratio should be 218 doctors for every 100,000 potential patients. Many patients, by choice or by neighborhood location, are seen by members of their ethnic group. It is therefore relevant to note that there are 241 White physicians per 100,000 White Americans, 875 Asian American physicians for every 100,000 Asian Americans, 69 Black physicians for every 100,000 Black Americans, and 45 Native American physicians for every 100,000 Native Americans. Libby, Zhou, and Kindig (1997) raise the important matter that these facts should influence medical school admissions.

Affirmative action admissions programs may represent the best available social policy to achieve a greater share of fairness and justice within a racially segregated society. These programs also provide the best means of educating future physicians to care for patients without regard to ethnicity. This is the ultimate color-blind goal we hope some day to achieve (Ludmerer 1999, 250). The rest of this book is devoted to exploring this and other arguments in favor of actively achieving this goal.

NOTE

1. President Lyndon Johnson's Executive Order 11246 established affirmative action requiring equal employment opportunity, relegating to the Department of Labor's Federal Contract Compliance activities to monitor hiring, retention, and promotion of women and minorities. These powers were expanded under the Nixon administration to require federal contractors receiving more than $50,000 annually to submit annual plans stipulating goals and timetables to reach them in hiring, training, and promoting minorities according to their availability in the pool of qualified potential applicants. Later the Equal Employment Opportunity Commission (EEOC) called for affirmative action by governments, and the Office of Education called for affirmative action by colleges (Welch and Grubel 1998, 12–14; Crosby and VanDeVeer 2000, 3–23). Medical school affirmative action was begun voluntarily in 1970, led by the AAMC in collaboration with the American Medical Association, the American Hospital Association, and the National Medical Association (Odegaard 1977, 23). This was done to remedy underrepresentation of minorities brought about by their exclusion, which required compensation with a goal to enroll 12 percent by 1975. Following the Bakke decision in 1978 affirmative action was also for the purpose of achieving diversity in the student body to enhance education for all students.

11. Affirmative Action

AT CORNELL

SINCE 1969, the Cornell University Medical College (now the Weill Medical College of Cornell University) has conducted a special summer program for minority students following their junior year, as one of its major institutional efforts to increase the enrollment of highly qualified minority students. The summer program has had a significant impact on every aspect of the minority program at Cornell. During my eleven-year tenure there, it was supported for six years by the Josiah Macy Jr. Foundation, partially for one year by the Robert Wood Johnson Foundation, for three years by the DHEW Health Career Opportunity Grants Program, and then directly by the institution. After I present the story of the first decade of general success in the Cornell minority recruitment and retention compared to the national yardsticks of success of such programs, I will delineate the specific contribution the special summer program made to this overall success.

From the outset I was convinced that only highly qualified minority applicants would be successful at Cornell, but there was little reason to expect such applicants to apply in view of a history of racial exclusion. From 1898 until the early 1970s only about eight U.S. Blacks and four foreign Blacks ever had graduated from Cornell. Only two American Blacks and two African Blacks had received degrees during the 1960s, even though approximately ninety students graduated each year.

In response to a growing national mood favoring affirmative action for underrepresented ethnic minority groups, concerned students and faculty at Cornell in the late 1960s urged the school to take a leadership role in this endeavor. In 1968 Cornell joined other leading U.S. medical schools in support of the targeted goal of increasing the enrollment of underrepresented minority medical students from a national level of about 3 percent to 12 percent by 1975 (Curtis 1971, 83–104). Nationwide, enrollments subsequently rose to 10 percent by 1974, but they declined to 8.7 percent in 1978. This figure obscures the fact that the experiences of individual medical schools were highly variable. The Cornell record of 10 percent or more minority admissions has been sustained through the present years but only because of special efforts.

DESIGN OF THE CORNELL SUMMER PROGRAM

The first Research Fellowship program for post-junior-year minority premedical students, not designed by me, was offered in the summer of 1969. It was completely different from all subsequent summer programs in several ways. In 1969, all ten minority students were Black, and all came from Hampton Institute, a Black college in Virginia. Several of the more able students were not even certain that they wanted to apply to medical school. In addition, the majority were either from Africa or the Caribbean with definite plans to return to their countries of origin.

It was immediately apparent to me that the summer program should not be confined to minority students from one school, nor limited to Black colleges, but rather should be directed toward the underrepresented ethnic minority groups from all major colleges and universities in the nation (Curtis 1971, 127–46). While participation in the summer program would undoubtedly be a mutual benefit for Cornell and the potential applicant, participation did not guarantee acceptance into the medical school. Minority applicants, including summer program students, applied in the same way as all applicants, and the same admissions committee acted on their applications. While participation probably would enhance an applicant's chances of being accepted by Cornell, it also would enhance his or her chances of being accepted by other schools. We also realized that there was no guarantee that applicants we accepted would choose Cornell.

As I outlined the beginning of the Summer Research Fellowship Program it was designed at first to be a collaboration between Hampton University, formerly Hampton Institute, and the Cornell University Medical College. Both Dr. Jerome Holland, president of Hampton and an illustrious Cornell alumnus, and Dr. John Dietrick, dean of Cornell's medical school, were members of the Cornell University Board of Trustees. The collaboration was informally and quickly planned during a weekend meeting of the board. While the collaboration undoubtedly expressed a benign paternalistic desire to promote minority medical school admissions, it became obvious to me during the first summer in 1969 that it showed little promise of success. It was during that summer that Dean Dietrick resigned and was replaced by Dr. Robert Buchanan. After discussing the matter carefully with Dr. Walter Riker and Dr. Walsh McDermott, the senior faculty of the medical school who were my strong support, my proposal was accepted that the Summer Research Fellowship program should be open to minority students from all colleges and universities, particularly those in the Northeast, from which Cornell's medical students usually came. This proposal was not viewed kindly by Dr. Jerome Holland or the Hampton faculty, and I received several offers of grant funding to limit the program to Hampton students. My preference prevailed, and that single decision made the program a success. Some further details of the beginning of the Summer Research Program can be found in my earlier book, *Blacks, Medical Schools, and Society* (1971, 83–104).

Since the summer of 1970 the program has had a uniform design and set of objectives. It has been offered to underrepresented ethnic minority premedical students completing their junior year of college who are citizens of the United States, have achieved a science grade point average of B minus or better, and who have strong recommendations from their premedical faculty advisers. Applicants wrote a one-page essay describing the development of their interest in a medical career and the benefit they expected from the summer program. These data were reviewed to determine which applicants would be interviewed either in person or by telephone. Each candidate was interviewed by two medical students who would assist in directing the program that summer. The student interviewers independently rated the candidate on a score of one to ten. In periodic supervisory sessions, in which all five of the medical student team leaders met with me as the project director, the top twenty-five candidates were selected. The program usually received three hundred applications, of which about one hundred applicants were interviewed and ranked from 1 to 30. The final twenty-five were chosen from this subgroup.

One of the principal aims of the program was to provide the student with an opportunity to do an independent study-research project under the sponsorship and supervision of a CUMC faculty member. This research fellowship experience occupied three full days a week and often a small amount of time on other days. A final written scientific report was required. Minority premedical students seldom have this kind of summer opportunity, which is available to nearly all very strong nonminority applicants, particularly children or friends of faculty or alumni.

In addition, the minority premedical student usually has had less exposure to the full set of career options available in the field of medicine and is less likely to have access to persons who can describe what the life of a medical student is like. Therefore, two days a week were set aside for other learning experiences. The students were given a sample course in cardiovascular physiology, taught by faculty members from both basic and clinical sciences, in which they were examined and graded. In the afternoons they were given a set of experiences that provided insight into the fields of public health and community medicine. One afternoon each week was spent visiting one of the special neighborhood-based community health programs located in a minority group community in the New York area.

Five first- or second-year minority Cornell medical students were employed full time as team leaders, to each of whom five summer program students were assigned. The medical student team leaders met regularly with their students and with me as the associate dean for minority affairs, in an effort to help all the program participants become successfully involved in all aspects of the program. In addition, each summer student was assigned to a third-year medical student volunteer, who met with the student weekly to discuss what is involved in caring for hospitalized patients and who took the student on ward rounds, usually to discuss a single patient. Most of these third-year students were nonminority students who volunteered. In sum, the minority premedical students were provided a set of life experiences aimed at equalizing their exploration of the field of medicine. The summer program offered the student friendly supportive personal relationships with both minority and nonminority individuals within the medical center and in New York City.

Admission to the summer program, including the experience of being interviewed, was in many ways a rehearsal of the medical school application process. Those who became program participants were given still further guidance on application procedures; all were encouraged to apply to Cornell, and all were advised on the specific schools at which they were most likely to be successful applicants. When I was responsible for the program, I met with each student several times and focused on how the students developed an interest in medicine, how they envisioned their future medical careers, and how they felt their careers would be influenced by their minority group status, all matters that many students at first found difficult to discuss.

At the conclusion of the period during which I directed this program (1969–81), it could be seen that students already were beginning to weigh the direction of their particular interests and whether they could handle the rigorous demands of medical student life. Since all students lived in the medical student dormitory during this ten-week period, they were afforded a preview of what they would encounter in the event they were accepted at Cornell. Their experiences would have been similar at many other schools and certainly would have enhanced their beginning medical education anywhere. Perhaps most unique was the experience of being one of a small group of highly selected minority premedical students and having the opportunity to form friendships that last a lifetime. It was our intent to leave them with the ideas that they could become part of the future medical leadership of the nation and that high levels of professional competence and social concern would be expected of them.

A DECADE OF MINORITY RECRUITMENT
AT CORNELL

Table 3 shows that in 1969 only twenty-five minority students applied to Cornell. Considerable effort was exerted by a small committee of nonminority students to obtain even that many applicants, since ordinarily fewer than a dozen applied. In the summer of 1969, when I went to Cornell to lead the minority program, no American Black students were enrolled in the medical school, one African Black had just graduated, and another was enrolled as a second-year student. From the small number of minority applicants, six were accepted, three enrolled elsewhere, and ultimately two entered the first-year class in the fall of 1969.

Beginning in 1970, and in each year through 1977, the first-year class included twelve to fifteen minority students. Growth in the minority applicant pool had to be stimulated by special efforts, of which the summer program was a major component. Specifically, six of the twelve minority students admitted in 1970 were Hampton graduates who had participated in the summer program the previous year. A number of them, as well as several of the other minority students admitted that year, had grade point averages and MCAT science subtest scores that were lower

TABLE 3. Cornell University Medical College Minority Applicants and Admissions, 1969–77

Year	Minority Applicants	Minority Admissions	Average Science GPA	Average Science MCAT
1969	25	2	2.10	500
1970	92	12	2.80	513
1971	151	14	2.95	536
1972	222	12	3.06	556
1973	292	13	2.98	565
1974	677	15	3.01	529
1975	565	15	3.25	585
1976	496	13	3.30	583
1977	552	13	3.21	601

Source: Data compiled by James L. Curtis during his tenure as associate dean.

than the average for minority students admitted in all subsequent years. The admissions committee paid attention to the students' motivation and excellent work habits—which we hoped would compensate for their relatively high academic risk. All but one of the six students ultimately graduated, although they encountered greater academic difficulty than subsequent minority enrollees. The admissions committee thought it advisable, however, that a critical mass of minority students begin their studies together, not only for mutual support, but also to mobilize more support from the institution. The presence of enrolled minority students was one of the most effective ways of recruiting additional ones.

The total applicant pool rose steadily for the first six years of the program before reaching a plateau, and average numerical indices of academic qualifications of admitted students steadily increased for the first seven to eight years. Not all this apparent improvement in quantity and quality of the minority applicant pool can be attributed to the summer program. All U.S. minority applicants were invited to apply to CUMC if their MCAT scores were at or above the fiftieth percentile, as indicated on the minority applicant register distributed to each medical school since 1969 by the AAMC Office of Minority Affairs. The MCAT science scores for minority students accepted at Cornell were more than a hundred points higher than the national average for all accepted minority students. For example, in 1973, Cornell's minority entrants scored 565; nationwide, the average science MCAT score of accepted Blacks was 472, while Mainland Puerto Ricans averaged 516, Mexican Americans, 521, Native Americans, 547, and Caucasians, 604.

Several important observations are helpful as a frame of reference when comparing nonminority and minority applicants and admissions to Cornell. There were approximately twenty-five hundred nonminority applicants each year for the years 1969 through 1974, and the size of the entering class was only 91 until 1973, when it was increased to 101. After the school joined the American Medical College Admission Service in 1974, the total number of applicants increased to the six thousand to eight thousand range, where it remained. In other words, despite a strong increase in the size of the minority applicant pool, the nonminority pool also expanded and remained ten times as large as the minority applicant pool. At the same time, the grades and MCAT scores of nonminority applicants improved decidedly.

In 1966 and 1967, before the minority program began, first-year science MCAT student scores for nonminority students admitted to Cornell were, respectively, 594 and 625. By 1971 and 1972, these nonminority scores had risen to an average of 643 and 642, respectively. In 1976 and 1977 they went up to 648 and 674. There was a sizable gap of between seventy-five and one hundred points on the science MCAT scores between the minority and nonminority first-year Cornell students.

There was also a substantial escalation of approximately fifty points among nonminority applicants to Cornell in the first decade of the program. Similarly, science MCAT subtest scores for accepted medical students nationwide increased on average from 577 in 1969 to 639 in 1977. Going back to 1959, the national average MCAT science score for all accepted students had been only 527.

A large national sample of students admitted during the 1950s and followed into the mid-1960s showed that science MCAT scores of 525 were associated with a dropout rate of 7 percent; scores of 625 with a dropout rate of 5 percent; scores of 725 with a 4 percent dropout rate (Johnson and Hutchins 1966). The Cornell admissions committee, like others, became increasingly selective in its admissions decisions during this period, for both minority and nonminority students.

A DECADE OF MINORITY RETENTION
AT CORNELL

After gaining admission to Cornell medical school the average minority student was presented with the challenge of competing with nonminority students who had received higher grades and MCAT test scores and had most likely attended the select colleges in the Northeast from which Cornell students are usually drawn. All Cornell medical students were graded and evaluated in the same manner (pass, fail, or honors). One might suppose it would have become easier for a weak student to drop out during the years under review (1970–78) because average grade point averages and MCAT scores were going steadily higher as described. A majority of the students voted to omit names from test papers; anonymous numbers were assigned to avoid favoritism in grading. Most of the basic science departments give norm-referenced tests that are graded on a curve, with the lowest scores automatically receiving fails regardless of what mastery of the subject they demonstrate. Unless the minority student exerted an above-average effort, he or she would be adversely affected by such a system. Nonetheless, this basically was the grading system in effect when the minority enrollment program began, and, because nobody wanted to lower standards, there was no push to change to a criterion-referenced grading system. In 1975 the medical school established new guidelines on promotion and graduation, in which students were automatically dropped from the medical school if they accumulated a certain number of failures, failed the same course twice, or weakly passed too many courses. The rules concerning the circumstances under which a student could be reexamined or repeat a whole year were also tightened.

Table 4 presents a summary of the retention success of minority students at Cornell in the decade from 1969 to 1978. It shows that from 1969 through September 1978, 12.3 percent, or 121 of the 980 students admitted to the first year, were minority students. Of that 121, 109 completed at least one and as many as four years of medical study at Cornell. Since Cornell is a four-year school, 62 members from six classes of minority students had been graduated in that affirmative action decade. The final column of table 4 shows that the 53 minority students enrolled in September 1978 included 2 who were a year behind their regular class placement. At that time there had been only 3 dropouts resulting from academic failure, which was largely conditioned by emotional problems except in one case; and 3 transfers, one of whom transferred to our graduate school of medical sciences for a more suitable research career, and two who had transferred to other medical schools from which they graduated. The minority retention rate was in the order of 97 percent, counting only 3 who were probably permanently lost to the study of medicine. It should be noted that as of September 1978, 7 of the 62 Cornell minority graduates had finished a year late because they were required to repeat a year. However, no students graduated more than a year behind the class with which they entered.

TABLE 4. **Cornell University Medical College Minority Enrollment and Retention, 1969–78**

Year	Total Entering Class	Total Entering Minority	Minority Graduates	Minority Transfers	Minority Dropouts
1969	91	2	0	1	0
1970	91	12	0	0	1
1971	91	14	0	0	0
1972	101	12	0	0	0
1973	101	13	1	1	0
1974	101	15	10	1	0
1975	101	15	14	0	1
1976	101	13	10	0	1
1977	101	13	13	0	0
1978	101	12	14	0	0
Total	980	121	62	3	3
Percent		12.3		2.5	2.5

Source: Data compiled by James L. Curtis during his tenure as associate dean.

~~These data can be contrasted with the experience of 862 nonminority~~ students admitted to Cornell in the same 1969–78 time period, of whom 773 had completed at least one year of medical school. Eight nonminority students transferred during this time period, and 9 dropped out. All others were either currently enrolled or had graduated. The nonminority retention rate is therefore between 98 and 99 percent. However, only 3 graduated a year late, substantially fewer than the number of minority students. Therefore, although the initial cognitive predictors gave the appearance of favoring the nonminority enrollees by a very large margin, the actual academic success rates were separated by a much smaller margin. This suggests that noncognitive factors are salient predictors of academic success for both minority and nonminority students admitted to Cornell, and probably most other medical schools.

Comparing these results with national averages (AAMC 1978, table 40, 4) at the end of 1974, 1975, and 1976, only 87 percent of Black students nationally were graduated or still enrolled, compared to 97 percent of nonminority students. The percentage of other minority students was intermediate. Retention rates for minority students at Cornell were 97 percent, and for nonminority students nearly 99 percent. A study of medical students admitted during the 1950s nationwide showed the following percentages of students graduated on time (i.e., four years after they were admitted): 88 percent of those with science MCAT scores averaging 525, 90 percent of those with scores in the 625 range, and 90 percent of those with scores in the 725 range (Johnson and Hutchins 1966). That same study showed that student success also was clearly related to the general level of support services provided by the institution's faculty and administration, particularly the student affairs staff (Johnson and Hutchins 1966, 1260). By any criterion, the retention of both minority and nonminority students at Cornell was at a high level.

ANALYSIS OF SUMMER PROGRAM PARTICIPANTS BY SUBGROUP

Table 5 shows the experience with CUMC summer program participants in the seven-year period from 1970 through 1977. The 1976 summer program students were not accepted into medical school until 1977, which explains missing numbers in the first two columns for the year 1977 in table 5. In this seven-year period the program admitted 143 of the 648 applicants (22 percent). Of the 143 participants, 132 (92.3 percent) were admitted to a medical school, 52 (36.4 percent) were accepted by Cornell, and 31 (21.7 percent) ultimately matriculated at Cornell. Only 11 of the participants failed to gain admission to any medical school.

The medical school acceptance rate probably is the best single measure of the fact that summer program participants were a highly selected group. Nationwide in the period 1974 through 1977, the percentage of nonminority applicants who were accepted ranged from 35 to 39 percent, while during those same years underrepresented minority acceptances decreased from 44 percent to 40 percent (AAMC 1978, 26). We cannot be certain that the summer program materially increased the proportion of program participants who would have been accepted by any school, but it very probably did account for their being accepted at a broader range of schools.

We can identify and further analyze the following subgroups of summer program students: Subgroup A ($N = 21$), who were accepted by Cornell but went elsewhere; Subgroup B ($N = 31$), who were accepted by Cornell and elected to come to Cornell; Subgroup C ($N = 80$), who were not accepted by Cornell but were accepted by another U.S. medical school; and Subgroup D ($N = 11$), who were not accepted by any school.

Table 6 summarizes some of the major differences among these various subgroups in terms of their science MCAT scores and science grade point averages. There was a significant pattern of difference in science MCAT scores in the subgroups of summer program students. Since admissions committees generally assume that high scores make an applicant more acceptable, the subgroups are not truly independent. Science grade point averages also show a significantly different overall pattern for the various

TABLE 5. **Cornell Summer Research Fellowship Applicants and Participants, 1970–76**

Year	Applicants	Participants	Participants Accepted to Any U.S. Medical School	Participants Accepted by CUMC	Participants Enrolled at CUMC
1970	30	16			
1971	44	20	13	7	6
1972	85	21	18	6	2
1973	96	22	20	8	5
1974	116	22	21	11	8
1975	137	22	22	5	5
1976	140	20	21	7	3
1977			17	8	2
Total	648	143	132	52	31
% of Total participants as of 1976			92.3%	36.4%	21.7%

Source: Data compiled by James L. Curtis during his tenure as associate dean.

~~subgroups A, B, and C, which are similar. Again, the science grade point~~ average is obviously not independent of membership in one subgroup or another. Students in subgroup A received acceptances almost everywhere they applied, while the other subgroups experienced decreasing acceptance rates. Clearly Cornell did not succeed in attracting minority applicants with the highest science grades and MCAT scores from the summer program; rather it succeeded in attracting the second level of minority applicants as they are defined by those numerical criteria alone. I will later probe more deeply into the extent to which these cognitive indices of ability carry real meaning in terms of actual academic performance.

All of the readily obtainable data on these several subgroups of summer program students were reviewed, including premedical colleges of origin, the medical schools in which they enrolled, what was known about their subsequent success in medical school, and the graduate medical education training programs they chose to enter. The numbers were too small to offer more than a hint of meaning to those latter queries, but we can report rather completely on the question of their initial colleges of origin and medical schools entered and graduated.

Subgroup A, the twenty-one who elected another medical school over Cornell, had come from the following colleges: Columbia or Barnard (four), MIT (three), Cornell (two), Harvard or Radcliffe (two), and one

TABLE 6. Science MCAT and GPA of Subgroups of Cornell Summer Program Students ($N = 143$)

	N	Science[a] MCAT	Science[b] GPA
Subgroup A	21	$N = 20$	$N = 21$
Accepted by Cornell		$X = 579.0$	$X = 3.09$
Preferred another school		$SD = 61.5$	$SD = .51$
Subgroup B	31	$N = 31$	$N = 31$
Accepted by Cornell		$X = 532.7$	$X = 2.94$
Enrolled at Cornell		$SD = 56.1$	$SD = .38$
Subgroup C	80	$N = 76$	$N = 78$
Not accepted by Cornell		$X = 496.8$	$X = 2.89$
Accepted at other U.S. school		$SD = 66.1$	$SD = .41$
Subgroup D	11	$N = 9$	$N = 11$
Not accepted		$X = 440.6$	$X = 2.52$
		$SD = 86.5$	$SD = .66$

[a]Overall difference among subgroups of summer program students is statistically significant at $p < .01$, by analysis of variance. All subgroups are significantly different from each other, by Newman-Keuls test.

[b]Overall difference among subgroups of summer program students is statistically significant at $p < .01$, by analysis of variance. By Newman-Keuls test, subgroup D is significantly different from the other subgroups, which are similar.

each from Penn, Yale, Princeton, Stanford, Wesleyan, Pomona, University of California, University of New Mexico, Fordham, and City College of New York. The medical schools they preferred over Cornell were Harvard (twelve), Columbia (three), Penn (two), and one each to the University of California at San Francisco, the University of New Mexico, Stanford, and Yale. All of these students can be considered to have graduated from medical school on schedule, including one who took an additional year to obtain a master of public health degree. Another student was a year late due to a voluntary decision to defer beginning her medical studies for a year, during which she worked on a special program at her college to enhance the preparation of minority premedical students. Specialties chosen through 1979 were medicine (four), surgery (two), psychiatry (two), and one each in family practice, pediatrics, and obstetrics and gynecology.

Subgroup B, the thirty-one who chose to enroll at Cornell, had come from the following colleges: Columbia (four), Cornell (four), Queens College (three), St. John's (two), Fordham (two), Hampton (two), and one each from Amherst, Brooklyn, Brown, City College of New York, Hofstra, Hunter, Lehman, New York University, Renselaer Polytechnic Institute, Smith, Virginia Union University, Wesleyan, Williams, and Yale. Only Hampton and Virginia Union University were Black colleges. All the other students were from colleges like those from which Cornell's nonminority students are ordinarily selected, although most of the schools were not quite as high in the prestige hierarchy. Of this group, two had graduated a year late as of the September 1976 review period, and all but one graduated. That student, who was on medical leave at the time of this review, later dropped out. Their chosen specialties for training through 1979 were medicine (eight), surgery (six), pediatrics (five), family practice (three), radiology (one), ophthalmology (one), and a straight medical research career (one). Their choices are compared with Cornell's nonminority students below.

Subgroup C, the eighty who were not accepted by Cornell but accepted by other U.S. medical schools, came from a broad array of colleges; but these students tended to come mainly from high-prestige schools either in the Northeast or elsewhere. Their undergraduate premedical colleges were Cornell (eight), Fordham (six), Yale (five), Columbia (four), Queens College (three), City College of New York (two), Hunter (two), Long Island University (two), and one each from the following: Albion, Antioch, Bard, Bates, Bowdoin, University of Claremont, Colgate, Emory, Fairleigh Dickinson, University of Illinois, Lehman, Macalester, Manhattanville, Mt. Holyoke, NYU, North Carolina State, University of Texas, Pembroke,

Radcliffe, Rutgers, Sarah Lawrence, Swarthmore, Trinity, Vassar, Vanderbilt, Xavier, and York College of the City University of New York.

The Black colleges contributed the following: Hampton (seven), Howard (three), and one each from Dillard, Fisk, Jackson State, and Talladega. Careful efforts were exerted to encourage summer program applicants from Black colleges. However, after relatively few of these students were accepted by Cornell, their participation waned. The medical schools these students attended were as follows: NYU (eight), University of Pennsylvania (seven), Columbia Physicians and Surgeons (six), Mt. Sinai (six), Boston University (four), Yale (four), Tufts (three), Howard (two), New Jersey College of Medicine (two), Meharry (two), Florida University (two), SUNY Syracuse (two), SUNY Downstate (two), Harvard (two), Emory (two), and one each to the University of Michigan, Duke, UC San Francisco, UCLA, SUNY Buffalo, Washington University, Michigan State, Northwestern University, UC San Diego, North Carolina, Cincinnati, Medical College of Virginia, Wayne State, Case Western, and Connecticut.

Of the eighty in this subgroup, we can report with certainty that six (7.4 percent) dropped out and at least fifteen (18.7 percent) graduated at least one year behind schedule. This suggests that the subgroups experienced progressive degrees of academic difficulty, going from subgroup A to B to C. Subgroup C's graduate medical education programs were in medicine (fifteen), obstetrics and gynecology (eight), family practice (three), surgery (three), and one each in ophthalmology, pediatrics, psychiatry, radiology, physical and rehabilitation medicine, and a flexible program.

Four of the eleven subgroup D program participants never applied to medical school, either because they did not believe they would like it or because they did not believe they would be accepted; the remaining seven applied but did not gain admission. Of this latter group, one applied to and was accepted at a medical school in the Dominican Republic after failing to gain entrance to a U.S. medical school. He was Black but of Dominican family background, fluent in Spanish, and also highly motivated. He found study abroad a positive and successful experience. Many of the students in this group came from excellent schools: Queens College (two), Wesleyan (two), and one each from Cornell, Bowdoin, CCNY, Dillard, Franklin College, Hampton, and Stillman College in Mississippi. However, even in this small list an overrepresentation of Black colleges is suggested, since Dillard, Hampton, and Stillman each contributed a student to this small subgroup. Although the low grade point average and low MCAT scores contributed to the failure of these students to gain entry to medical school, these numerical indices were not their only weakness.

From intimate knowledge of these students I gained the impression that they would not have become successful medical students. Two of them clearly seemed to lack ability, despite strong motivation and good work habits; most of the others were uncertain in their motivation, work habits, maturity, emotional stability, or self-confidence. A distinct impression was that the summer program served these students well in the degree to which it helped them more realistically assess their strengths, weaknesses, interests, and desires, or chances of successfully pursuing medical careers.

COMPARING CORNELL MINORITY STUDENTS WITH AND WITHOUT SUMMER PROGRAM EXPERIENCE

Table 7 summarizes data on the performance of minority students admitted to Cornell, with or without their having had the benefit of the summer program. This was a stringent and clear-cut test of the overall impact of the summer program. Minority summer program enrollees who entered Cornell had significantly lower grades and lower science MCAT science scores than minority students who had not been in the summer program. The sixty-four nonsummer program Cornell minority students had science grades and MCAT scores almost identical to the twenty-one subgroup A summer students who had been accepted by Cornell but chose another school. Table 7 further shows that the thirty-one subgroup B summer program students outperformed their sixty-four peers by measures of

TABLE 7. Comparison of Minority Students Admitted to Cornell with and without Summer Program Experience

	N	Science MCAT	Science GPA	Total Number with Zero Class Failures	Total Number with One or More Honors
With summer program	31	$N = 31$	$N = 31$		
	(32.6%)	X = 532.7	X = 2.94	14	23
		SD = 56.1	SD = .38	(45.0%)	(74.0%)
Without summer program	64	$N = 61$	$N = 64$		
	(67.4%)	X = 577.1	X = 3.19	25	38
		SD = 67.9	SD = .45	(39.0%)	(59.0%)
	95				
Total	(100.0%)				

Statistically significant findings:
 Comparing difference in science MCAT: $t = 3.34, p < .001$
 Comparing difference in science GPA: $t = 2.83, p < .01$

Source: Data compiled by James L. Curtis during his tenure as associate dean.

~~subsequent academic performance. Despite statistically significant lower~~
MCAT scores and science grades on entrance, the thirty-one summer program students accumulated proportionately more honors and fewer failures than their sixty-four minority classmates at Cornell who lacked the summer program experience. All midterm and final grades in all courses are included, regardless of whether the course was taken one or more times. It is important to note that the four summer program students who obtained five or more failures had MCAT scores ranging from 475 to 605; the twelve other minority students with five or more failures had scores ranging from 485 to 635. Only one of the thirty-one summer program students had as many as eight failures; seven of the other 64 minority students had between eight and twelve. These results primarily are a record of academic performance during the first and to a slightly lesser extent second year since at Cornell, as in most medical schools, it is uncommon for students to do failing work in the third or fourth years. What we observed was that students who had our summer program experience for ten weeks in the year prior to beginning their medical studies at Cornell achieved sufficient emotional and social advantages that the subsequent quality of their academic work was improved. Combined with that, the CUMC decision to admit that student in the first place was probably more soundly based, as it rested on a more complete appraisal of the applicant's noncognitive and cognitive strengths. For all practical purposes, the summer program student is actually given the experience of being a special student at Cornell for a brief trial period, and it is not surprising that it pays off. Several years of sustained effort were required to evaluate this aspect of the program.

Looking over the experience of those first few years, one can conclude without doubt that several of the minority students who were most unhappy with their choice to come to Cornell would have been able to make that prediction had they spent ten weeks there beforehand. Problems can be predicted if a student has not been able to make a single durable friendship from among his peers, medical students, and faculty after ten weeks at the medical center. Considering that a student may be unhappy in one school and yet thrive in another, it is demonstrably better both for the student and for the medical school if they prefer each other from the start. Because of this, a student with several options should always be encouraged to attend his or her first choice.

Other factors that possibly could differentiate the two groups of Cornell's minority students did not seem to be relevant. Men and women were equally divided in the two groups, the summer program students were 64 percent male, our nonsummer program students 75 percent male; summer students were 71 percent Black with the remaining Hispanic, while the nonsummer program minority students were 70 percent Black.

Cornell's minority students who had not gone through the summer program also came primarily from colleges and universities in the Northeast, were much more widely dispersed, but seemed to represent the same prestige range: Queens (four), CCNY (four), Brooklyn (three), Harvard (three), NYU (three), Amherst (two), Columbia (two), Fordham (two), Lehman (two), MIT (two), and one each from California State–San Bernardino, Carnegie Mellon, Colorado, Delaware, Haverford, Hunter, Indiana, Marist, Montclair, New York Institute of Technology, Renselaer, Rutgers, Stanford, Stevens Institute of Technology, St. Johns, St. Louis University, Swarthmore, Trinity, University of Bridgeport, Kentucky, Maryland, Penn, Rochester, Wagner, Wesleyan, Wellesley, Williams, and Yale. Only two of these students were from Black colleges, Clark College and Morris Brown, both in Atlanta.

Another way of comparing the success of the thirty-one summer program students to the other sixty-four minority students was by looking at the numbers from each group who experienced special problems such as dropping out, transferring, or graduating a year or more late as of September 1978. The summer program group had no dropouts or transfers from 1971 through the September 1978 cutoff date. The summer program student who went on medical leave and dropped out later in the next year should be considered to have fallen into the group of students with problems. Two additional summer program students graduated a year late. Therefore a total of three (9.7 percent) fell into the special problem group as we have defined it.

In contrast, until September 1978 there were two dropouts, two transfers, and eight students who graduated a year late among the sixty-four nonsummer program minority students. Every one of these twelve (18.8 percent of the 64) students experienced considerable emotional stress that caused substantial wear and tear on the faculty and administration as well.

National Board Medical Examination test results provided another means of comparing the summer program and non–summer program minority students. While Cornell does not require its students either to take or to pass any part of the National Board for promotion to the third year or to graduate, more than 99 percent take these examinations voluntarily. Part 1 is given at the end of the second year. Comparing twenty-eight summer program students with fifty non–summer program students, the non–summer program students passed only one subject, behavioral sciences, with a higher score, 446.7 compared to 404.8. This was significantly higher ($p < 0.4$). In all other subjects the scores for the two groups were not different, and their average total scores were not significantly different (447.7 for the summer program students compared to 456.2 for the non-summer program students).

Recalling that initially there was a significant difference in favor of the nonsummer program students, both in their MCAT science scores and science grade point average, this initial difference seems not to have been sustained. In those same years the Cornell nonminority students' part 1 scores ranged from a low total average score of 517.8 in 1975 to a high of 581.4 in 1973. This illustrates the fact that despite wide year-to-year fluctuations, the minority and nonminority average scores were still separated by an obviously significant fifty to one hundred points, just as was found in their initial science MCAT scores.

Part 2 National Board examinations for seventeen summer program students showed no difference either for any specific subject or for the total average score, compared with thirty nonsummer program minority students (average total scores actually were 431.4 and 426.0 respectively). Again, Cornell's nonminority students achieved average scores that ranged from a low of 531 to a high of 553, significantly greater by a hundred points or more. However, the nonminority students' initial MCAT science scores, in the high 600s on average, were in a considerably higher percentile range than either part 1 or part 2 of the National Board examinations scores, although all of those examinations are scaled to go up to 800 points. It is, of course, difficult to determine what the average National Board scores would be, either for minority or nonminority students at Cornell, had they known they would be required to pass them in order to be promoted or graduate. A passing score for part 1 is only 380, and for part 2 it is 290, considerably lower than the scores of minority or nonminority Cornell students.

Internship training program choices for the thirty-one summer students, compared to the other sixty-four minority students, are interesting but without any statistically significant differences. There were only nineteen summer program graduates of Cornell from 1975 to 1978, compared to thirty-one non–summer program minority graduates. Bearing these proportions in mind, note that their Graduate Medical Education Year 1 (GME-1) training program choices respectively were medicine (6 and 16); surgery (6 and 7); pediatrics (2 and 4); family practice (2 and 1); obstetrics and gynecology (0 and 1); radiology (1 and 0); psychiatry (0 and 2); ophthalmology (1 and 0), and medical research (1 and 0). Fifty-two percent of the non–summer program students chose medicine, compared to only 32 percent of the summer program students. The large number of summer program students who entered surgery is partly explained by the observation that 4 of the 6 who made that choice did so in 1978 alone. Among Cornell's nonminority students who graduated in 1978, 24.4 percent entered surgery, compared to 17.4 percent as their average for the preceding three years. The department of surgery had positive appeal for more than an average number of students in that entire class. One of the chief residents in surgery that year was an extremely able Black who won an award as best teacher on the house staff. Also important was the fact that one of the former summer program students, who had strong leadership potential and chose surgery, also may have had more than ordinary influence on all the minority students in his graduating class.

In a similar vein, all three of the minority students from Cornell who selected family practice residencies during this period were Puerto Rican. (There were only five Puerto Rican graduates in that time.) It will be worth observing in the future whether or not the increased group cohesion that provided peer support among the summer students, and to some extent among minority students generally, may have the unintended effect of diminishing the individuality in their GME-1 program choices. This is only a speculation, but it is probably of some substance.

Internship choices for Cornell's 264 nonminority graduates in the 1975–78 period were as follows: medicine was most popular, with 61 percent; surgery, 19 percent; pediatrics, 9.5 percent; family practice, 3.4 percent; psychiatry, 2.2 percent; obstetrics and gynecology, 0.6 percent; and others negligible. These data suggest that compared to national averages (Task Force on Graduate Medical Education 1980, 166), Cornell sent almost twice the usual proportion into medicine, slightly more into surgery, and far below average percentages into family practice, psychiatry, obstetrics and gynecology, or the support specialties. Combined minority student choices (fifty in number), for purposes of comparison were medicine, 44 percent; surgery, 26 percent; pediatrics, 12 percent; family practice, 6 percent; psychiatry, 4 percent; obstetrics and gynecology, 2.0 percent; and others negligible. Even with these small numbers it seems that significantly fewer minority graduates, compared to Cornell's nonminority graduates, went into internal medicine ($p < .04$); other differences are within the range of chance fluctuation.

Geographic locations of the chosen internship training programs cannot be reliably compared because of small numbers. No apparent differences were noted in comparing the summer program minority students with their minority peers. Comparing all minority graduates with their nonminority Cornell classmates does suggest a different pattern of choices, which may in time reach statistical significance. The differences are in the expected direction: minority graduates more often chose programs located in large inner-city ghetto neighborhoods. For example, in the New York metropolitan area alone, Harlem Hospital, which is predominantly Black, drew five minority graduates and three nonminority graduates during this 1975–78 period; Montefiore, which is predominantly Puerto Rican, drew four minority and one nonminority Cornell graduates; Kings County Hospital in Brooklyn received two minority graduates and no nonminority graduates; and Martland Medical Center in Newark received one minority graduate and no other. The trend will be an important one to follow, because several able minority graduates definitely have preferred training programs in minority neighborhoods over opportunities to enter programs in more prestigious locations, and in more high-status academic settings. It is also my speculation that a few nonminority Cornell graduates selected training programs in the inner city at least in part because of positive associations with their minority classmates.

TWENTY YEARS OF PROGRESS

Taking a longer-term view, I note that between September 1970 and September 1991, 317 minority students matriculated at Cornell University Medical College. Of that number 231 graduated, 14 withdrew, 2 transferred to other schools, and 70 were enrolled at the cutoff point for this analysis. This yielded an overall retention rate of 94 percent (Bruce Ballard, personal communication, 1991).

Table 8 compares medical school enrollment by race and/or ethnicity at

TABLE 8. Enrollment at Cornell and Other Medical Colleges, by Race and/or Ethnicity, 1991

Race and/or Ethnicity (%)	CUMC	United States
White	66.9	71.8
Asian or Pacific Islander	15.1	14.4
Black or African American	10.1	6.6
Mexican American/Chicano	2.7	1.8
Puerto Rican (Mainland)	2.4	0.7
Other Hispanic	1.7	1.7
American Indian/Alaskan Native	0.4	0.4

Source: Data for U.S. from Section for Student Services, Association of American Medical Colleges, October 21, 1991. Totals do not sum to 100 because it was not possible to categorize some of the enrollees.

Cornell with all medical colleges in the United States for September 1991. Here it can be seen that Cornell actually had fewer White students than the national average, and it had larger numbers of Asian or Pacific Islanders, Blacks or African Americans, Mexican Americans, and Mainland Puerto Ricans, while the percentages for other Hispanics and Native Americans were the same. This shows that minority recruitment efforts at Cornell have been quite successful, a fact that is demonstrated in a different way in table 9, which shows the percentages of the applicant pools of all underrepresented minorities and the percentages who enrolled both for Cornell and the United States during the years 1987–91. The very active recruitment program is a national one.

Table 10 shows the top five specialties chosen by CUMC minority graduates from 1988 to 1991 compared with other CUMC and U.S. minority and nonminority graduates. Here it can be seen that Cornell minority graduates exceeded their peers from other schools in their selections of internal medicine, ophthalmology, and psychiatry, while fewer chose pedi-

TABLE 9. Percentage of Minority Applicants and Enrollees at Cornell and All U.S. Medical Schools, 1987–91

Year	CUMC		United States	
	Applicants	Enrollees	Applicants	Enrollees
1987	11.5	11.9	10.6	9.0
1988	11.6	16.8	10.8	9.0
1989	12.0	14.9	11.3	9.3
1990	10.2	14.9	10.8	9.2
1991	10.4	14.9	10.8	9.8

Source: Data for United States from Section for Student Services, Association of American Medical Colleges, October 21, 1991.

TABLE 10. Top Five Specialties at Cornell and All U.S. Medical Schools, 1988–91 (%)

	CUMC		United States	
	Minority[a]	All Others	Minority[a]	All Others
Internal medicine	30.5	26.0	15.0	16.2
OB-GYN	10.2	6.4	14.2	7.6
Ophthalmology	10.2	3.7	2.0	3.1
Psychiatry	10.2	11.1	6.6	5.3
Pediatrics	8.4	9.9	11.3	9.2

Source: Data for United States from Association of American Medical Colleges Survey on Practice Plans for 1990 U.S. Graduates.

[a]Refers to underrepresented minority.

atrics or obstetrics and gynecology. Their selection of internal medicine exceeded that of all other groups.

Specialty choices of the 231 minority graduates of Cornell for the years 1974 through 1991 were as follows: internal medicine, 81 (35.0 percent); pediatrics, 23 (9.9 percent); obstetrics and gynecology, 20 (8.6 percent); psychiatry, 17 (7.3 percent); general surgery, 16 (6.9 percent); ophthalmology, 10 (4.3 percent); anesthesiology, 10 (4.3 percent); family practice, 8 (3.4 percent); orthopedics, 8 (3.4 percent); urology, 6 (2.6 percent); radiology, 5 (2.2 percent); pathology, 4 (1.7 percent); otolaryngology, 3 (1.3 percent); neurosurgery, 3 (1.3 percent); preventive medicine, 3 (1.3 percent); medicine and pediatrics, 2 (0.8 percent); dermatology, 2 (0.8 percent); neurology, 2 (0.8 percent); clinical pharmacology, research law, undecided, and nonresponders to recent inquiries, 8 (3.1 percent).

THIRTY YEARS OF AFFIRMATIVE ACTION
PROGRESS AT CORNELL

Let's now take an even longer-term view. Information provided by Dr. Bruce Ballard, Cornell Medical School's associate dean for student affairs, shows the thirty-year record (September 1970–2000) of recruitment, enrollment, retention, and graduation of underrepresented minority students (URMs). In that period 471 URM students were matriculated; 376 graduated; 64 are currently enrolled, not including 6 M.D.-Ph.D. students in the Ph.D. segment of training, and also not counting 2 medical students currently spending a full year in research, and 1 M.D. student on leave but in good standing. A total of 19 students withdrew, of whom 2 enrolled in another medical school to complete their study. Three students transferred elsewhere to complete their medical studies. The overall retention rate is 94.4 percent.

For graduating classes in the years 1998, 1999 and 2000, of the total 303 graduates, 58 graduates, or 19 percent, were URM students. Their minority group membership was American Black, 32, or 55 percent; Mainland Puerto Rican, 12, or 21 percent; Mexican American, 11, or 19 percent; and Native American, 3, or 5 percent.

Their choices of postgraduate training programs were medicine, 18 of the 58; general surgery, 10; and another 2 each went into urology or orthopedic surgery; emergency medicine, 6; obstetrics and gynecology, 6; family practice, 5; pediatrics, 7; psychiatry, 1; and pathology, 1.

Cornell has a special interest in producing graduates who will pursue a career in medical research. Of special interest is the career of Dr. Mae Jemison, a Black American woman who graduated from the Stanford University

School of Engineering in 1977, also as a major in Afro-American Studies. She was admitted to the Cornell University Medical School and received the M.D. degree in 1981. She did not participate in the summer program for minority students. On graduating from medical school she had general medicine postgraduate training at the Los Angeles County Hospital's University of Southern California division. We made every effort to have her continue postgraduate training at our institution. After two years in private practice she spent several years in West Africa as a medical officer in the Peace Corps.

Seeking a new challenge in 1987, she joined the NASA astronaut program, and, because of her background in engineering and medicine, she was selected for the shuttle team as science specialist when the successful flight was launched in 1992. After earning a Ph.D. degree from Lincoln University, she retired from NASA in 1993 to pursue a career in technology and science education, heading her own consulting firm, which has developed telecommunication systems for several West African nations. Currently she is a professor of environmental studies at Dartmouth, where she directs the Jemison Institute for Advancing Technology in Developing Countries (*New York Public Library* 1999, 278).

MINORITY FACULTY AT CORNELL

Minority faculty numbers and representation in the medical school administration have also shown progress. Dr. Bruce Ballard's position is associate dean for student affairs and equal opportunity programs and is chiefly responsible not only for minority student recruitment but also for advising and counseling all students in all four years. Dr. Ballard, a graduate of Yale and then of the Columbia University College of Physicians and Surgeons, succeeded me in my position at Cornell in 1980 and since expanded his role on the dean's staff. Dr. Ballard also holds a faculty appointment as associate clinical professor of psychiatry.

Another minority member of the medical school dean's staff is Dr. Carol Storey-Johnson, a graduate of Yale and a participant in our summer program. She graduated from the Cornell Medical School, having been elected to AOA, the scholastic honor society, and trained at the New York Hospital in internal medicine. She became the director of ambulatory medical clinics, and for two years she was associate dean for academic programs. In the past year she has been named senior associate dean for education programs; three associate deans report to her in areas of admission, student affairs, and academic affairs. Dr. Storey-Johnson is an associate clinical professor of medicine.

Hiring and retention of minority faculty continues to be one of the most difficult areas for all medical schools. In 1999 U.S. medical school faculty totaled 89,717, of whom Blacks represented 2.8 percent, Mexican Americans 0.4 percent, Mainland Puerto Ricans 0.8 percent, and Native American 0.1 percent. Essentially these proportions have not changed, except for women, who in 1979 represented 15 percent of total medical school faculty; in 1999 they represented 38 percent. Data for 1977–78 indicated that total full-time faculty at medical schools were 2.5 percent for underrepresented minorities, but no data were given on how many of these were at Howard and Meharry, the two predominantly Black schools. The contribution of these two schools must have been great inasmuch as in 1967–68, underrepresented minorities were the identical 2.5 percent (Higgins 1979, table 4, 74; table 5, 45). The sensitivity of these matters is shown by the fact that between 3.6 percent of male faculty and 2.8 of female faculty failed to respond to the AAMC survey on gender and ethnicity (AAMC 2000, 316).

When the author joined the Cornell faculty in 1969, there was only one other Black faculty member in a full-time faculty position, a woman associate professor of obstetrics and gynecology. Since that time there has been a dramatic increase in the minority faculty representation at the Weill-Cornell Medical College. In the year 2001 there were a total of forty-three full-time faculty members, eight of whom identified themselves as Hispanic, of which two are Puerto Rican, and thirty-five who are Black. Their faculty ranks as follows: two full professors, fourteen associate professors, twenty-two assistant professors, four instructors, and one senior research associate (Bruce Ballard, personal communication).

Cornell's success is a result of sustained effort: currently five separate programs are targeted at talented minority students at the high school and college levels and also at students with special interest in careers in medical research and academic medicine ("Advancing Minority Student Recruitment" 1996).

III. Civil Rights

IN HEALTH CARE

SLAVERY AND RECONSTRUCTION

AFTER THE SOUTHERN SLAVES were set free by the Emancipation Proclamation, their health status and health care declined sharply. This paradox becomes easy to understand if we recall that slaves were valuable property because the fruit of all their labor and all of their children were assets of the master. The state of medical knowledge in the antebellum South was of course on a low order. Large plantations commonly employed a White physician and usually had a hospital or infirmary with older slave women as nurses or attendants (Morais 1969, 11–20; D. B. Smith 1999, 11–12), but we should bear in mind that only 2 percent of slaves lived on plantations with 250 or more slaves while the overwhelming majority lived with families holding 15 or fewer slaves (Fogel and Engerman 1974; Fogel 1989, 178–79). The enslaved population increased from close to 700,000, or 25 percent of the nation's total population in 1790, to close to 4 million in 1860. Some 250,000 were brought in illegally after the end of slave importation in 1808, with growth in the slave population thereafter due to natural increase (*New York Public Library* 1999, 32). The average slave woman during the child-bearing years gave birth to slightly more than nine children (Fogel 1989, 14, table 4; among Caucasians, "American marriages yielded, on average, about eight live births . . . and half of these children lived to maturity" [115]). This was roughly twice the number of children born to a slave woman in Trinidad, most likely due to the shorter fertility span and higher death rates of slaves in Trinidad. Generally slaves fared worse on the large sugar plantations in the tropics.

Newborn babies were small in size, most of them probably weighing less than 5.5 pounds, making them vulnerable to early death from diarrhea, dysentery, whooping cough, and a variety of respiratory diseases. Malnutrition probably was a major cause of the low birth weight and continued in the early years of life, accounting for the fact that death rates for slave children were twice those of White children (Fogel 1989, 143). The excess death rate for children under five accounts almost entirely for the higher mortality rate for slaves as compared to Whites.

That adult slaves in the United States enjoyed relatively good health is indicated by the fact that life expectancy of slaves and Whites was similar after age twenty. Analyses of cotton picking and other fieldwork schedules suggest that pregnant women worked with little letup until the last weeks of their pregnancies, returned to work after a month, and were at full schedules by the fourth month, suggesting that their babies were weaned early (Fogel 1989, 146).

Computations based on 1850 census data indicated that the average death rate due to pregnancy among slave women aged twenty to twenty-nine was just "one per thousand . . . not only low on an absolute scale, it was also lower than the maternal death rate experienced by southern White women." Fogel and Engerman (1974, 123) go on to note that the infant mortality rate in 1850 was 183 per thousand for slaves, while for Whites nationwide it was 146 per thousand, or 20 percent lower. Most of this difference vanishes when we note that the infant mortality rate for southern Whites in 1850 was 177 per thousand, "virtually the same as the infant death rate of slaves" (124). These figures would suggest that life in the South generally was not as favorable.

The rapid influx of European immigrants into New York, Philadelphia, and Boston in the period 1820–60 greatly exceeded job opportunities available to them, resulting in high rates of crime, homelessness, poor health, and alcoholism. "Life expectancy at birth for persons born in New York and Philadelphia during the 1830s and 1840s averaged just twenty-four years, six years less than that of Southern slaves" (Fogel 2000, 58, 59). Fogel and Engerman (1974, 258–64) maintained that the abolitionists had deliberately exaggerated the brutality of slavery, understandably to rally opposition to the inhumane and degrading nature of the institution. In the process of emphasizing its cruelty, Blacks inadvertently were depicted as a group of totally demoralized and victimized incompetents. Thus the Black slave was seen as inferior for reasons of social oppression, but nonetheless as inferior as though it were genetically induced. It was that distortion of history that constitutes a racist attack on Black people, making it appear that they are beyond hope for betterment. By calling attention to the strength of Black people, even under enslavement, in terms of physical health, labor productivity, and as skilled artisans and managers of plantations, Fogel and Engerman did not intend to glamorize or excuse the injustice of slavery, but simply to set the facts straight. Even in the strength and stability of their family life, the slaves were more successful than commonly supposed.

W. M. Byrd and L. A. Clayton, in their comprehensive medical history of African Americans, paint a gloomier picture of the health of Blacks in the antebellum South (Byrd and Clayton 2000a). Primarily citing the work of T. L. Savitt, they point out (285) that overall mortality rates for slaves in rural or urban communities were almost one and a half times higher than for Whites (Savitt 1978). Byrd and Clayton showed that slaves were extensively used as research subjects by White southern physicians like J. Marion Sims, often referred to as the father of gynecologic surgery for his discoveries in 1830 to 1850 on the repair of vesicovaginal fistula and his invention of surgical instruments used in obstetrics and gynecology. Similarly, Crawford Long used slaves extensively in his 1842 discovery of ether anesthesia for patients undergoing surgery.

With the end of slavery, White Southerners no longer had a vested interest in the welfare of Blacks. In the immediate postemancipation period, many planters tried to reconstruct their plantation work gangs on the basis of wage payments, but the freedmen rejected these incomes, which would have exceeded "by more than 100 percent" their real earnings as slaves. Once free, slaves rejected forced labor in gangs because of its "nonpecuniary disadvantages" (Fogel and Engerman 1974, 237–38). As a free agricultural worker farming on a sharecrop arrangement, with no protection against exploitation, the freedmen were on a rapid downhill course that brought them back essentially to a condition of hostile reenslavement.

Life expectancy for slaves in the 1880s and 1890s declined by 10 percent compared to the quarter century before the Civil War. Their diet deteriorated; sickness rates by the 1890s generally were 20 percent higher; they were driven out of the skilled crafts that they had previously dominated; and they were barred from membership in labor unions. Only with World War II did this trend reverse itself, and since then decade by decade there has been a reduction in differential life outcomes between Blacks and Whites, which revives a sense of possible improvement (Fogel and Engerman 1974, 261). Fogel and Engerman agree with (1974, 261) Gunnar Myrdal, who, in *The American Dilemma,* observed that the surviving system of color caste in some limited respects was a more precarious economic arrangement than slavery. As David Barton Smith reminds us (1999, 21–24; see also Hoffman 1896), near the end of the nineteenth century a number of commentators claimed that because Blacks had an infe-

rior constitution, which made them vulnerable to diseases like tuberculosis, and were prone to sexual promiscuity (resulting in venereal disease),
drug abuse, and alcoholism, they would probably become an extinct race
within a few decades. Social Darwinism was becoming widely accepted in
that era; survival of the fittest was the way it was and should be. A dramatic worsening of the health status of Blacks was seemingly confirmed by
the census in 1870, 1880 and 1890; in 1890 for the first time the Black
birthrate was lower than the White (Byrd and Clayton 2000a, 411). A
prominent health care statistician, Frederick Hoffman, predicted that the
Black race would be extinct by the year 2000, and his work convinced
most insurance companies that Blacks were uninsurable.

In the antebellum census of 1850, the life expectancy of slaves was 36
years, 12 percent below the average 40 years for White Americans. In 1890,
life expectancy for Whites was 47.6 years, for Blacks 33 years, a 30.7 percent difference—illustrating how much less support the social system was
giving to Blacks as free men and women (Fogel and Engerman 1974,
125–26). Fogel (1989, 179) summarizes studies on family stability among
slaves and concludes that it was closely related to plantation size. For the
43 percent of all slaves who lived on plantations where there were fifteen
or fewer slaves, only one-third of the children were raised in two-parent
families; on larger plantations, two-thirds of slave children lived in families headed by both parents. The general family pattern was that the father
was head of the house. We should note that in the 1990s two-thirds of
Black children were in single-parent homes, as compared to 24 percent in
1960 (Jaynes and Williams 1989; *New York Public Library* 1999), reflecting
a relatively recent decline in family structure that has disproportionately
affected African Americans.

SEPARATE BUT EQUAL

If Congress had acted favorably on the radical Republican proposal to give
each slave family forty acres and a mule as startup capital after the Civil
War, debilitating poverty could have been prevented in ensuing generations. The Homestead Act of 1862, passed before the end of slavery in 1865,
gave 1.6 million White families up to 162 acres each if they agreed to live
on and farm what had been public land. In the same year the Morrill Act
established the land-grant colleges, which were almost exclusively for the
benefit of Whites. Subsequent amendments provided additional funds in
1890 and again in 1907 (see J. O. Smith 1987, 19–61, who details land give-
aways to Caucasians from the colonial period; and Cross 1984, 495–526,
esp. 516–17). Smith points to these as examples of economic, educational,

and civil rights for Whites, guaranteed by law and birth, while rights for Blacks depended historically on the kindness and good grace of their adversaries and competitors. In a highly competitive and adversarial society, this is not good. For example, seventeen so-called Black colleges were set up by states; these were required under later revisions of the Morrill Act to provide separate but equal schools for Blacks. As of 1916, not one of them provided college-level courses leading to a bachelor's degree; all were boarding schools teaching elementary and high school subjects (Jones and Weatherby 1978, 102–3).

When the slaves were freed, they were left penniless and homeless, their plight so desperate that in 1865 Congress empowered the president to appoint a commissioner to direct the Freedman's Bureau, to look out for their welfare and education. Blacks had a driving need to own land, and the commissioner had authority to lease unoccupied tracts of land and sell it to ex-slaves after a period of three years. Rents paid by the freedmen, who were not allowed to have more than forty acres each, amounted to $400,000, an amount that practically paid for the Bureau's operation during the first years. A Freedmen's Saving and Trust Company was established by a group of philanthropic supporters who arranged for it to be chartered by the federal government and for two-thirds of its assets to be in government securities. Headquartered in Washington, D.C., there were twenty-seven branches situated primarily throughout the South. The bank remained strong from 1865 until the early 1870s despite strong opposition from Whites who resented the presence of banks within their states that they could not control. Southern Whites gained control with a bill that Congress approved allowing changes in the Board of Trustees membership, which reduced the proportion of deposits invested in federal government bonds, allowing other notes and real estate mortgages as collateral. As J. O. Smith states, this opened the bank's vault to predators, and within three years the hard-earned savings of many newly freed men were lost (1987, 108–9). While the Freedmen's Bureau controlled 800,000 acres of land in 1865, by 1868 the amount was reduced to fewer than 140,000. The Bureau was phased out in 1872, leaving only the philanthropy of church denominations to aid in setting up Black schools and colleges. The Freedmen's Bureau's medical department had set up more than ninety hospitals and dispensaries in the South but by 1868 closed all except the largest and strongest one, Freedmen's Hospital, on the grounds of Howard University.

Both Howard University Medical School and Meharry Medical College were established under the auspices of the Freedmen's Bureau. Morais

(1969, 39–58) discusses the histories of these two institutions. Howard opened in 1868, with the stated objective of admitting Blacks or Whites, although it was "primarily intended to train colored doctors." One of their first eight students was White. Of the five initial faculty members, one was a Black physician who had been educated in Canada. At first classes were held only in the late afternoon and evening, not only because students had to hold jobs during the day, but also because the White faculty members were also on the faculty of the medical school at Georgetown University. They encountered great pressure to resign from their association with Howard at the risk of losing or being demoted from their Georgetown appointments. They persevered, and Howard gained a good reputation and membership in the Association of American Medical Colleges.

Unlike Howard, Meharry was established in 1875 solely for the education of Negro doctors, first as a part of Central Tennessee College supported by the Freedmen's Aid Society. It became a freestanding school in 1915. Unlike Howard, which was funded by the federal government, Meharry was financed privately. Its first building, to accommodate the first dozen students, was built with funds from the five Meharry brothers, White businessmen who were showing their gratitude to Blacks who had helped them in their early careers.

Between 1869 and 1900 ten Black medical schools were established (Watson 1999, 23–43). Flexner's 1910 report on the nation's medical schools concluded that, of the seven Black schools then in existence, only Howard and Meharry were strong enough to warrant continued support. Flexner's endorsement made a medical school eligible for a portion of the $100,000,000 made available by the Rockefeller General Education Fund to establish a stronger scientific base for medical education. Only rarely did a medical school in the East, such as Harvard, Yale, or Penn accept a Black student. Midwestern schools, like Michigan, Indiana, and Northwestern accepted Blacks only a bit more frequently. Thus, as of 1895, there were 365 Negro physicians, only 27 (7 percent) of whom had graduated from White schools. In 1905, of the 1,465 Black doctors, 213 (14.5 percent) were graduates of White institutions. From 1905 essentially until the affirmative action programs began in 1970, the unofficial quota of Black graduates from predominantly White medical schools remained the same (Morais 1969, 60).

It is important to note that Flexner had a limited view of the role of Blacks as physicians, believing they could do more good as public health sanitarians in rural communities than practicing as surgeons in the cities. He further believed that Black physicians would only treat Black patients,

who would be better off with well-educated Black physicians than poorly
educated White ones (Morais 1969, 230).

AN EQUAL RIGHT TO HOSPITAL CARE:
THE TUSKEGEE VETERAN'S
ADMINISTRATION HOSPITAL

Blacks were largely excluded from the American hospital system until the
legal end to most racial barriers in the 1960s, as is illustrated by the events
surrounding the opening of the Tuskegee Veteran's Administration Hospital, established in Alabama in 1923 specifically to care for Black veterans.
Black people have had a long struggle to gain equal access to hospitals, either as patients who need care or life-saving treatment, or as attending
physicians with privileges to admit and care for their sick patients, or professional nurses. Like many important and shameful racial stories, this one
has seldom been exposed to public review (Morais 1969, 112–16).

After fighting to make the world safe for democracy, many soldiers who
returned from World War I required hospital care for mental and physical
disabilities they sustained during military service. The Veterans' Bureau,
finding hospital facilities around the nation inadequate to meet the needs
of veterans, built hospitals to provide suitable care. Black veterans were excluded outright from these hospitals or forced to accept beds only on segregated wards. The problem was particularly acute in the southern states,
where three-fourths of the four hundred thousand Black veterans lived at
that time.

Around this same time Booker T. Washington in effect advised Blacks
not to agitate or struggle for their political and civil rights, but rather to
remain in the South and make an accommodation to the separate and
second-class status imposed upon them. He believed that by quietly promoting their vocational and economic development, they would eventually
become accepted as equal Americans. Washington's philosophy was anath-
ema to W. E. B. DuBois and his more militant Black colleagues and White
collaborators. DuBois and others founded the National Association for the
Advancement of Colored People in 1910. Their goal was to free Blacks from
the restrictions of color caste and to gain for them every single privilege of
first-class citizenship. Even Robert Moton, president of the Tuskegee Institute—founded by Booker T. Washington, who died in 1915—was sym-
pathetic to this newer and more self-respecting point of view.

Pressure from Blacks for more decent and equal care continued until
the Harding administration sought Moton's advice and assistance. In response to Harding's request for help, Tuskegee gave the United States gov-

ernment five hundred acres of land, a mile from their campus, as a site for the construction of a veterans' hospital to be used for Blacks from any part of the nation. It is difficult to imagine that the president of the United States would have to accept the advice of and then a gift from the president of a Black college in the South before decent hospital care was grudgingly extended to Black war veterans.

With the gift came the stipulation that the hospital would be staffed by Black physicians and nurses. Built at a cost of $2.5 million, the six-hundred-bed hospital was completed in 1923. To the surprise of Moton and other Blacks, the Veterans' Bureau appointed not only a White physician as head of the hospital, but also a full staff of White physicians and White nurses. Black nurses' aides were appointed in order to limit the direct contact between the White nurses and the Black male patients. When Blacks insisted that Black professionals replace the Whites, the Ku Klux Klan marched, held nighttime demonstrations, and made death threats. But Blacks persisted, and in July 1924 a Black physician was made director. By the end of the 1920s, Black physicians, including those with specialist training, ran the entire hospital. In the 1930s no other Black hospital in the country, including those associated with Howard and Meharry, could equal the facilities, staff, budget, or residency training programs of the veterans' hospital at Tuskegee. (A detailed history of the political struggle to gain Black control of this hospital, and of the decision to locate it at Tuskegee, has been provided in exemplary scholarship by Vanessa N. Gamble [1995; see esp. 70–104]).

By the end of the 1930s Tuskegee's hospital had grown to fifteen hundred beds, about half dedicated to psychiatric patients, while the rest were for general medical and surgical cases. By that time some of the northern states had begun to admit as patients their Black veterans who required hospitalization and to treat them more equally.

Given the presence of highly trained Black specialists in medical and surgical fields, it remains a source of amazement that the Tuskegee syphilis experimental study was conducted there, in Macon County, Alabama. Begun in 1932 and lasting until 1972, it was perhaps the longest experiment in withholding treatment from human subjects in medical history. The study, conducted by the United States Public Health Service, with the full collaboration of Tuskegee Institute, involved following the untreated course of syphilis in 399 Black men from that rural area who had the disease and who were given no treatment even after the 1940s when it was known that penicillin was an effective cure. Researchers compared their clinical course with another 201 Black men who did not have the disease.

As David Barton Smith (1999, 25–28) points out, this reflects badly on the sense of medical ethics and fairness on the part of Black and White professionals. "It was not a secret experiment conducted by rogue researchers. Outside professionals regularly reviewed the project's protocols. More than a dozen publications were generated and were widely read . . . even after the county medical society had become a predominantly black body in the late 1960s the project continued to receive full support including the referral of patients to the project's control group" (26). Tuskegee Institute's administration and its private hospital located on campus (John A. Andrew Hospital) cooperated fully with this research, allowing its facilities to be used in medical evaluations of these men. The Veterans' Administration hospital did not cooperate as fully, although their staff pathologist performed autopsies on the more than one hundred men who died in the course of the research, and sent organ specimens to the National Institute of Health for definitive study (Jones 1981, 122–50).

My speculation is that neither Black nor White middle-class and educated physicians could put themselves in the place of those uneducated Black farmhands who had syphilis. The public learned of the project in 1972, and it was halted quickly; but despite the fact that the federal government has paid more than 10 million dollars in an out-of-court settlement to surviving participants and their families and heirs, it has left a lasting monument to the power of indifference to the mistreatment of uninformed and vulnerable Black men.

AN EQUAL RIGHT TO HOSPITAL CARE:
LOUIS T. WRIGHT AND
HARLEM HOSPITAL, 1919–52

John Knowles (1973) made the point that the hospital system is a barometer of our social values and belief systems at any given time. Much of our voluntary hospital system was developed by religious denominations, with hospitals specifically labeled as Protestant, Catholic, or Jewish and with special service missions for their own groups. At first these hospitals were built and financed by wealthy contributors from their religious constituencies. The public charity hospital system had the residual responsibility of caring for the sick poor who were otherwise left out of the voluntary-sectarian hospital system. However, these hospitals were generally closed to Blacks by law in the South, and by custom and practice elsewhere. Meanwhile, modern urbanization of the American population was simulating the development of large city hospitals. The medical profession's need for teaching and research facilities strengthened the growth both of the large voluntary-sectarian hospitals and of large public charity hospitals.

One of these large public charity hospitals was Harlem Hospital in New York City; and the story of the battle to open it up for Black staff is most revealing (Corwin and Sturges 1936; Morais 1969, 117–28; Reynolds 2000). Following World War I, the Black migration to New York City had surrounded Harlem. By the 1920s, many newspaper stories began to recount the inadequate, incompetent and unfair treatment accorded to the large number of Black patients crowding into Harlem Hospital.

Dr. Louis T. Wright was the first Black physician appointed to the medical staff of Harlem Hospital, and he is the leading figure in this powerful story. Both his father, who died young, and his stepfather were Black physicians and prominent leaders in the Atlanta community. In 1897, his stepfather, William Fletcher Penn, was the first Black to graduate from Yale University Medical School. Although he was first in his class, Penn was unable to find postgraduate training in the East, so he completed an internship at Freedmen's Hospital in Washington, D.C. He then founded a Black hospital in Atlanta and established an interracial practice. In 1925 Penn accepted the position of chief of surgery at the Veterans Administration Hospital at Tuskegee, where he remained until his death in 1934.

Louis T. Wright graduated fourth in his class from Harvard Medical School in 1916, but also could not find training at a teaching hospital and had to go to Freedmen's Hospital, where he performed brilliantly. He volunteered for military service and, while serving in France, worked side by side with White physicians and nurses on surgical wards, where he soon was put in charge.

In 1919, Dr. Wright was the first Black physician appointed to the medical staff of Harlem Hospital, though at the lowest possible rank. The White hospital director of Harlem Hospital was immediately denounced for making the appointment and forced to transfer to another city hospital. Four White physicians resigned from the Harlem Hospital Center's staff rather than work with a Black physician. Another prominent White surgeon resigned from the staff after a nursing school to train Black nurses was established in 1923. He refused to have a Black nurse assist him in the operating room. By 1929, of sixty-four physicians and surgeons on the staff of the hospital, only seven were Black. Not until the following year was the staff reorganized, and in 1930 the salaried staff to care for inpatients included nine Black physicians. In that same year another seven Black physicians were in the outpatient department, and nine Blacks were appointed as interns. Nineteen dentists were added in 1931.

A study prompted by the National Association for the Advancement of Colored People concluded in 1935 that Harlem Hospital was important because it was the only hospital in the country where Black physicians were on the same footing as the White members of the staff and enjoyed exactly the same privileges. Moreover, it was one of the very few hospitals, outside of the so-called Black hospitals, that admitted Blacks as interns. That is why all that pertained to Harlem Hospital assumed a national importance.

Nevertheless, only four Blacks applied for internship in 1933, and many Black physicians in the Harlem community expressed heated criticism of Dr. Wright, claiming that he favored the Black graduates of predominantly White medical schools over the graduates of Howard or Meharry. Indeed, for at least another decade, a lively controversy existed within the Black medical community in Harlem concerning the wisdom of establishing an all-Black hospital, completely controlled and staffed by Blacks for Blacks, a movement that Dr. Wright vigorously opposed and that never gained wide support. Into the 1930s and 1940s Harlem Hospital continued to provide internship training for many able Black physicians graduating from all the nation's medical schools. Its racially integrated professional staff achieved a level of excellence—especially in its surgical training program, led by Dr. Wright—that brought it recognition throughout the national medical community (see Maynard 1978, for an excellent account by the surgeon who succeeded Dr. Wright as head of the Harlem Hospital Center Department of Surgery).

In 1931, data from the American Medical Association, and from a special study by the Jules Rosenwald Fund, showed that 122 hospitals, distributed throughout twenty-eight states and the District of Columbia, would accept Black patients. Of these, the only hospitals with a two-hundred-bed or larger capacity were tax supported: two of these were federal and two were city hospitals. Another two state hospitals, a county and a city hospital, had bed capacities between one hundred and two hundred. Seventy percent of the hospitals for Blacks only were of less than five-hundred-bed capacity, and half of them had fewer than twenty-five beds each. Of all these Black hospitals, the AMA had approved internship training programs in fourteen, although many were pitifully weak. Two of the strong and well-established hospitals with all-Black patients accepted only White men as interns: Grady Hospital in Atlanta, associated with Emory University School of Medicine, and St. Phillips Hospital in Richmond, associated with the Medical College of Virginia (Corwin and Sturges 1936).

Against that historical background we can see that many gains had been made by 1956, when Reitzes (1958, 329–48) studied the racial pattern of medical care in fourteen major urban centers of the United States and found that the presence of a Black hospital in a given city influenced, usually negatively, the degree to which a racially integrated pattern of hospital care was being achieved (333). Such a hospital encouraged self-segregation. On the other hand, it could be argued that the presence of Black hospitals merely reflected the extent to which entrenched racial segregation in that city had forced the development of a separate hospital system, in lieu of none at all. Predominantly Black hospitals were absent in the six cities that had the highest degree of integration as measured by an index of the percentage of Black physicians having appointments at predominantly White hospitals. These cities were New York, Philadelphia, Los Angeles, Indianapolis, Boston, and Gary, Indiana. Detroit, where Black hospitals were relatively unimportant, was the seventh most integrated, followed by cities with important Black hospitals: St. Louis, Chicago, Kansas City, Washington, D.C., Atlanta, Nashville, and New Orleans (Reitzes 1958).

An exception to the self-segregationist trend was Washington, D.C., where two very strong Black institutions, the Howard University College of Medicine and its affiliated teaching hospital, Freedmen's, nevertheless produced Black leaders who pressed for racial integration of the hospital system in our nation's capital (Reitzes 1958, 338). In 1956 Washington ranked third among cities in number of Black physicians, with 224; New York was first and Chicago was second. But regarding the number of board-certified specialists, Washington was first, with fifty-eight; Chicago with forty-two was second; New York with forty was third. Medical integration, however, had begun seriously in Washington only in 1948. That was the first year that Black physicians were accepted as members of the attending and resident staffs of the Gallinger Municipal Hospital (now the District of Columbia General Hospital); Children's Hospital opened up its training program in 1955. Black physicians were not accepted as members of the Medical Society of the District of Columbia until 1952, the same year that Hadley Memorial Hospital first opened its doors to Black patients and staff. The Health Department desegregated its programs in 1953. In 1954, for the first time, a Black physician was appointed to the staff of the teaching hospital of George Washington University. In 1955, George Washington University Medical School admitted its first Black student; by that year Georgetown had accepted several, but none had enrolled. Most of these gains came as the result of steady integrationist pressure from the Black faculty members and alumni of Howard University (Reitzes 1958).

THE END OF RACIALLY SEPARATE HOSPITALS

The United States Supreme Court did not outlaw racially segregated hospitals until 1964, ten years after the legalized end of public school segregation. Following World War II, the Hill-Burton Hospital Construction Act of 1946 provided the means by which $2 billion in federal funds were spent building an improved hospital system for the nation. Out of deference to southern custom, and specifically to obtain the strong support of Senator Lister Hill of Alabama, localities were allowed to build "separate but equal" hospitals, or wings of hospitals, for Blacks and Whites, as long as the state plan nominally provided for equal hospital care for both races. This was modeled on "separate but equal" language in the Morrill Land Grant College Act, which financed inferior educational institutions for Blacks. Not surprisingly, these federal funds had the effect of escalating the building of new edifices for racial separatism. By 1949, as many as 214 hospitals built with Hill-Burton funds were racially separate in whole or part, and 4 had been built exclusively for Blacks. In 1962 and 1963, civil rights proponents in the Congress, led by Representative John Dingell from Michigan and Senator Jacob Javits from New York, introduced bills to require hospitals that received Hill-Burton funds to admit Black patients and to give staff privileges to Black physicians. These legislative efforts failed. It was, moreover, the opinion of chief legal counsel for DHEW that, while patients could not be denied admission to those portions of so-called nondiscriminatory facilities built with Hill-Burton funds, such facilities were not required to grant staff privileges to Black physicians, nor was it required that Blacks be accepted into their postgraduate or other training programs (Morais 1969, 180–82).

In 1963 a group of Black physicians, dentists, and patients sued two hospitals in Greensboro, North Carolina, for refusing to accept Blacks as patients or professionals. This dramatic story is covered in wonderful detail by David Barton Smith (1999, 91–114; see also Morais 1969, 180–98). These litigants argued that the "separate but equal" provision of the Hill-Burton act be declared an unconstitutional denial of their Fourteenth Amendment equal protection rights. In that same year, in the case of *Simpkins v. Cone Memorial Hospital,* the federal district court in North Carolina decided against the plaintiffs, but on appeal the Fourth Circuit Court reversed this decision and granted the relief sought by the Black plaintiffs. Throughout the land, Blacks were jubilant about this victory.

Interestingly, the *Journal of the American Medical Association* gave the case scant acknowledgment, mentioning it in a column on Washington news ("Miscellany—Segregation" 1963). The defendant hospitals immediately appealed the case to the Supreme Court, which refused in 1964 to hear the appeal, thereby letting stand the decision of the Fourth Circuit Court of Appeals. Again the matter was treated lightly by *JAMA* ("Washington News" 1964). *JAMA* explained that, while the equal protection clause only protects persons from unequal government actions, the voluntary hospital had received Hill-Burton funds in an amount judged by the court to be sufficient to bring them under this constitutional requirement. Cone Memorial had received $1.2 million in federal funds but had refused to give Black doctors and dentists staff privileges, although they had admitted a few Black patients. Long Hospital, another party to the legal action, had received $2.9 million and was closed to Blacks either as patients or as professional staff. The reader was left to ponder whether it was a correct interpretation that those voluntary hospitals were considered to be acting as government agencies. There was no reference to any medical or moral issue. This was not the end of AMA activity, however. It became known, and was reported by Montague Cobb in the *Journal of the National Medical Association,* the Black medical journal, that an AMA representative appeared before a congressional committee requesting legislation to exempt private or voluntary nonprofit hospitals that received federal funds from being considered as public or governmental agencies (Cobb 1964). No such legislation was ever introduced. In fact, later in 1964, after a ten-year court contest, Black physicians won a still more decisive case, bringing about substantially more equal hospital rights. In the case of *Eaton v. Walker Memorial Hospital,* a hospital in Wilmington, North Carolina, was required to cease all racial exclusionary practices even though it was not a recipient of Hill-Burton funds as such; other funds from the city and state government had gone to that hospital, entitling Blacks to equal hospital treatment.

Title VI of the Civil Rights Act of 1964 mandated nondiscrimination in federally assisted programs on pain of losing their funds, requiring federal agencies to promulgate regulations translating those requirements into action. The regulations of DHEW that implemented that act explicitly prohibited racial discrimination in patient admissions, as well as any separate or different treatment on account of race, nor could there be racial discrimination in the selection of interns, residents, nurses, student nurses, and other trainees, or in granting professional staff privileges or appointments.

The 1965 Medicare and Medicaid amendments to the Social Security Act brought a still greater amount of federal funds into the financing of hospital care. We should note that while the American Public Health Association and the American Nursing Association supported passage of Medicare and Medicaid, the American Medical Association not only vigorously opposed these laws financing medical care for the elderly and the poor but tried unsuccessfully to have the Black National Medical Society fight it (D. B. Smith 1999, 115–28). Civil rights compliance was energetically pursued by DHEW in those early years, with five hundred staff members assigned to review the policies and practices of eight thousand hospitals, many of them being credited with changing their racial behavior. Unfortunately, by the mid-1970s the federal political climate and administration had changed, and on-site inspections or the actual use of a fund cutoff was widely viewed as an empty threat. In fact the rules had been rendered more obscure and vague, and both staff and budget to enforce civil rights compliance had been reduced to symbolic proportions.

As David Barton Smith explains, the Office of Civil Rights within the then Department of Health, Education, and Welfare (DHEW) was in 1977 given responsibility for enforcing Title VII prohibitions against denial of equal rights to Blacks, but actually much more compliance staff time and thought were devoted to school desegregation than to health services. When DHEW was reorganized under the Carter administration, the Health Care Financing Administration (HCFA) gained authority over Medicare and Medicaid programs, which should have provided more leverage over health care providers. Providers, however, effectively nullified this authority. As one staff member said, "HCFA was a captive of the industry in the late 1970s. . . . We tried for years to get HCFA to include race data. . . . The department never took it on and we never got anywhere" (D. B. Smith 1999, 183–85). When DHEW was transformed in 1980 to become the Department of Health and Human Services, a separate Office of Civil Rights was created, but with the election of Ronald Reagan in November 1980, civil rights enforcement was a dead issue. Even during the Clinton years, the Office of Civil Rights had only one-third as many staff members as in 1979 and had been transformed "from a central driving force into an increasingly isolated, decaying part of the federal bureaucracy" (D. B. Smith 1999, 187).

HEALTH CARE ORGANIZATION RESPONSE TO THE DESEGREGATION MANDATE

David Barton Smith (1999, 317–19) has presented the most telling analysis of the ways in which the health care delivery system responded to this newly mandated desegregation environment. Fundamental changes were to be expected: There has been a shift away from federally monitored acute hospital care to more state monitored long-term nursing home care, and a great increase in the number of diagnostic and treatment interventions performed on an ambulatory basis as well as increased home-based care. Smith maintains that many of these changes had the intent of minimizing Black and White patients having to share rooms or to sit together, and to increase the likelihood that they would be standing up together while they were receiving care. Black patients are at a disadvantage because of the dearth of privately sponsored ambulatory services and long-term care facilities in their neighborhoods, all of which have forced their greater reliance on teaching hospitals and clinics. All things considered, however, much less rancor and hostility have been associated with hospital desegregation than with school desegregation.

Young physicians still learn to practice on poor and ethnic minority patients, and when they finish their training, they set up practice in suburban areas. Even if they remain in the city, they accept few poor patients because of Medicaid's low reimbursement rates and burdensome paperwork. The chance that a Black patient's cholecystectomy would be performed by a surgery resident in 1962 was 2.5 times higher than a White patient's; in 1972, this likelihood for Black patients had increased to 4.3 times (D. B. Smith 1999, 234). In medical schools that have affiliations with both public general hospitals and private hospitals, the schedules usually are arranged to ensure that the public hospitals are heavily staffed by residents.

Without doubt, however, profound changes for the better occurred following strict Title VI antidiscrimination enforcement in the Medicare program. Health care utilization by Blacks improved dramatically, although disparities still exist. Mortality rates continue to favor Whites by a wide margin in almost all outcome measures, and Blacks receive fewer of the more expensive and technologically complicated procedures.

Another marked difference is that Black-owned and Black-operated hospitals have disappeared. Between 1961 and 1988, seventy Black hospitals closed or merged with historically White facilities either because of financial pressure or a need to meet high standards to continue to attract Black patients (D. B. Smith 1999, 195). Regional Health Systems Planning activity in the mid-1970s, and passage of the Medicare Prospective Payment System in 1983, forced these health care system changes, which would appear to benefit Black patients.

Organizations respond to policy changes. Medicare equal opportunity requirements may have reduced within-hospital segregation—but they may also have stimulated the creation of new proprietary hospital chains, the relocation of hospitals from the inner city to the suburbs, and a change in the mix of acute and chronic patients receiving care within the same hospitals. An index of segregation represents the proportion of Blacks and Whites who would have to move to create an equal distribution of the two groups, with 1 meaning that 100 percent would have to move. In fiscal year 1993, there were a total of 11 million Medicare acute care hospital discharges, 84 percent White, 10 percent Black, 3 percent other, and 3 percent unknown; the index of segregation was roughly .53 for the nation as a whole (D. B. Smith 1999, 219). Significantly, the segregation indices for states in the Midwest and Northeast were much higher than for states in the Deep South, where hospitals had desegregated more than other regions. Many southern states' hospitals have indices of .20 to .30, while the Northeast and Midwest range from .40 to .70. Just as public schools in the South currently are less racially segregated than in the North, East, or Midwest, the same holds true for hospitals. De facto segregation now carries more force than de jure segregation.

Hospital practice has changed nationally in ways largely influenced by legal requirements for desegregation. Length of stay has been shortened to the point where ours are the shortest among all developed nations in Western Europe and in Japan, despite the fact that our per capita hospital costs are the highest in the world. Further, over the past thirty years many diagnostic and treatment services have been shifted from inpatient to ambulatory clinics, and many more hospital rooms are now private or for two patients only, another expensive practice not seen to such an extent anywhere else in the world. Smith believes this is often done in part to keep Black and White patients separated.

Even more basic changes are at least in large part racially driven (D. B. Smith 1999, 318). Nursing homes were not held to strict Title VI antidiscrimination standards. Coincidentally, between 1963 and 1973, the number of nursing home beds doubled. A 1981 Institute of Medicine study concluded that Blacks are discriminated against in nursing home admissions, in part because of reimbursement arrangements: nursing home administrations prefer patients whose families can pay the out-of-pocket higher rates; they will keep their certified bed capacities low to avoid increasing state Medicaid budgets, which actually pay for the majority of patients. High and frequently arbitrary selection decisions will therefore tend to diminish chances for a Black to be admitted, and nursing home administrators completely control admission decisions. In years past, many chronically ill Black patients stayed longer in acute hospitals, but the demands for short stay have begun to curtail this practice.

Private physician practice patterns also escaped Title VI antidiscrimination monitoring because physician groups opposed such close scrutiny of office private practice and the increased paperwork it would require. Further, the cost of reviewing physician practice medical records would have been insupportable as well as nonproductive. Indeed, only a small fraction of physicians participate because of the lower rates of reimbursement by Medicaid and Medicare compared to private insurance. With the advent of the managed care medical market, Medicaid, Medicare, and private employer health plans will increasingly force all physicians to begin to enroll all patients who have any third-party coverage. The intimate character of the relationship between the physician and patient is being radically redefined because of restrictions of freedom of choice imposed by managed care.

Residential racial segregation continues to be a fact in most metropolitan areas of the United States. David Barton Smith (1999, 287) reminds us that White Medicaid recipients are geographically diffused throughout residential areas and therefore are more easily absorbed in private practice physicians' caseloads. Black Medicaid patients, recognizing that they are forced to rely more on teaching hospitals and clinics, bring a greater legacy of distrust and fear that they will be receiving inferior and less personalized care. Patient privacy seems to be less assured, with the expected but unfortunate result that sensitive problems such as alcoholism or substance abuse are less likely to be discussed, diagnosed, or treated with professional compassion and are less likely to result in referral for expert and peer group management. These are among the serious ongoing problems that will continue to be a hurdle in our national effort to reduce health care disparities between Black and White Americans. Black physicians still find that about 87 percent of their patients are Black, while only 7.4 percent of White physicians' patients are Black (Health of the Disadvantaged 1977). Improving the health outcomes for Black patients will, of course, depend on improving their access to high-quality, professional, personalized medical care from Black and White physicians, all of whom should be trained to be proud of fulfilling their professional calling to serve all who are in need.

SUMMARY

During slavery the health care and health status gap between Whites and Blacks was less than at any time since Blacks became free. Also during slavery Blacks were more fully employed than at any time since. Beginning with Reconstruction, the health status of Blacks declined; it has only begun to improve with gradual advancement in our national economy and with Civil Rights activities that followed World Wars I and II, culminating in the civil rights legislation of the 1960s after Martin Luther King's assassination.

De jure hospital segregation ended in the 1960s and 1970s, creating greater but still unequal access to hospitals for Blacks as patients, staff physicians, resident trainees, and nurses. All-Black hospitals have practically ceased to exist, and we should apply sustained pressure to desegregate the hospital system nationwide.

Managed care will present serious challenges to equal treatment of Blacks.

PART II

iv. Geographical Distribution

OF MINORITY RESIDENTS

IN THE PRECEDING CHAPTER I described the process by means of which Black Americans gained access to hospitals as patients and also as professional staff, beginning first in racially segregated settings such as the veterans' administration hospital in Tuskegee, Alabama, and the Harlem Hospital Center. Both of these developments came in the aftermath of World War I as a result of demands of the Black community.

In part 2 I outline the entry of African Americans into mainstream hospitals, which occurred in the context of sweeping social changes in American social structure following World War II. Among the major driving forces for these changes were the democratization of higher education, the increased wealth of new science and technology, and the breaking down of social class and religious barriers, which had limited the size of the American middle class. College enrollments in the nation increased from two million in 1946 to eight million in 1970 (Ludmerer 1999, 188). While Black Americans enjoyed some of these gains through the GI Bill of Rights, they were still largely handicapped by being confined to a segregated rather than mainstream educational pathway; even mortgages guaranteed by the GI Bill still largely confined them to segregated neighborhoods with inferior public schools. No longer did a bachelor's degree reflect special knowledge; graduate students in those same 1946 to 1970 years increased from 120,000 to 900,000. Similarly, an M.D. degree giving one the right to practice general medicine after a year of rotating internship was no longer a sign of professional competence. Beginning in the late 1940s and swiftly setting a new pace, postgraduate training leading to specialty board certificates became the new standard of competence for physicians. Hospitals had increased in number, supported by governmental funding, and teaching hospitals offering approved residency training positions increased from 5,796 in 1940 to 46,258 in 1970 (Ludmerer 1999, 181–83). The American public was demanding more medical care, and of a higher quality, especially when financial barriers to care were significantly removed in the late 1960s by the passage of Medicare and Medicaid governmental funding, both of which generously provided not only for patient care but financed residency training programs as well.

Between 1956 and 1980 the number of United States medical schools increased from 84 to 127, enabling first-year enrollments to double, going from 8,000 to 16,590. Medical school enrollments and annual graduation rates could not keep up with the residency training positions offered: in 1958 U.S. medical schools graduated 6,861 students, but 12,325 residency training positions were offered by teaching hospitals that year. A special Surgeon General's consultant group in 1959 advised that the nation's health could not be protected unless medical schools increased their annual graduates from 7,400 to 11,000 by 1975. Federal funding made this possible, and the targeted increase was met.

In all of these vastly expanded opportunities Black Americans were only minimal beneficiaries because color caste confined them to segregated settings. Slowly the color line was melting, as shown by the new way that public and private hospitals desperate for staff had begun to hire Black nurses. A signal event occurred in 1951, when the National Association of Colored Graduate Nurses, which had been founded in 1908, disbanded. Leaders in that organization and in the predominantly White American Nursing Association agreed that all nurses should belong to a single national group, and that the thirty or so Black nursing schools also could go out of business because almost all of the 1,152 nursing schools nationwide were already accepting qualified applicants regardless of color (Morais 1969, 199; D. B. Smith 1999, 42–44).

The medical establishment was slower to change, but significant changes occurred for some previously excluded groups. With more resident training positions and more medical students entering and graduating, quotas against Jews and Catholics, at that time excluded minorities, disappeared (Ludmerer (1999, 206–7), but in the 1950s and 1960s no positive steps were taken to recruit women or members of other minority groups. It was not until affirmative action programs began in 1970 that women and minorities were admitted to medical schools in greater numbers and therefore could gain acceptance to postgraduate training teaching hospitals.

The shortfall of medical school graduates led to a huge and sudden influx of foreign medical graduates (FMGs): from 1950 to 1959 alone foreign medical graduates in the nation's residency training programs increased from 2,072 to 9,457. By the late 1960s, 30 percent of all residents were

FMGs, and even then 20 percent of all residency training positions went unfilled. It was this shortage of U.S. graduates in matching the huge increase in residency training positions that forced our hospitals to import foreign medical graduates for almost ten years before minority groups (primarily Black) and women graduating from U.S. medical schools were available to be recruited and accepted beginning in the 1970s.

As a sign of how much Black medical school graduates were on the outside looking in, McLean observed in his introduction to Reitzes's *Negroes and Medicine* that in 1947 only eight graduates from Howard and Meharry combined were accepted for residency training in any predominantly White hospital in the country; by 1956 the number had increased only to forty-six (Reitzes 1958, xxvi). In 1947, with specialty training as the new standard, only 93 Blacks nationwide were board certified specialists, a number that grew to 190 by 1952 and to 320 by 1957. This was less than 1 percent of all U.S. board-certified specialists. McLean saw clearly that all American medical schools should actively recruit qualified Black students and that all residency training directors should welcome them. Clearly both doors had to be opened: to all medical schools, and not just Howard and Meharry, which enrolled 85 percent of Black graduates in those years, and to all postgraduate training programs that were importing physicians from abroad or leaving positions unfilled.

Even now, Fitzhugh Mullan (2000) believes, a case can be made to increase the number of physicians we graduate from medical schools. For the past two decades we have continued to graduate only about 16,000 new physicians a year, but we still have about 22,000 residency positions to be filled, even though we turn away at least as many qualified medical school applicants as we accept. As a nation we have become chronically dependent on foreign medical graduates to fill these vacancies, and we allow them to remain here in the hope that they will practice in underserved areas. A sounder plan, in Mullan's view, would be for us to develop creative ways of graduating more minority and nonminority physicians from this country willing to make career commitments to practice in underserved areas.

OVERVIEW OF THE COMPARATIVE STUDY

In part 2 of this book I present data on two thousand minority medical school graduates and two thousand nonminority medical school graduates in the five-year period 1973 through 1977, comparing geographical location and area of residency specialist training they selected in those years, and indications that some hospitals more than others in various regions of the nation were actively recruiting or affirmatively enrolling minority medical school graduates. Important differences are observed between these two groups of young physicians, who in different ways are making important professional contributions to our national life, health, and welfare.

In 1975 and again in 1976 I made unsuccessful attempts to obtain data from all student affairs deans in United States medical schools on the GME-1 training program choices of all their graduates, along with an identification of the ethnic group membership of each graduate. This initial approach was via mailed questionnaire. Failing to get a sufficient set of data, I used another approach, which resulted in almost complete samples.

All GME-1 placements matched through the National Internship and Residency Matching Plan (NIRMP) are routinely sent to student affairs deans at all medical schools. These alphabetized lists were used as a starting point for assembling our samples for the years 1973, 1974, 1975, 1976, and 1977. The Matching Plan works as follows: Medical students apply to a number of hospital training programs, ranking the hospitals by their numerical choice or preference. Hospitals rank the applicants by order of preference in the same fashion. The actual internship placement is decided by the highest mutual match of the student and the hospitals. The five-year period used for this study was 1973–77. In general, these students entered medical school four years prior to their year of graduation. Lists of all medical school graduates nationally are given in alphabetical order, with coded numbers identifying the student's medical school and the hospital chosen, and a code for the specialty training program in which that student matched. However, no information as to whether a student is a member of a minority group is available from these lists, nor other NIRMP databases.

In order to identify each student's minority group membership, several student research assistants and I went back to the Medical Minority Applicant Registries (Med-Mar) distributed by the AAMC annually since 1969. These registries contain the names and minority group self-designation of all minority medical school applicants who choose to be so identified at the time they take the MCAT. Almost all members of our minority sample were identified in that way. Since this register did not exist in 1968, it could not help us to identify minority students who graduated in 1973; those using the 1969 register would ordinarily not graduate until 1974.

Another method employed to identify minority applicants was to consult the published newsletters of all National Medical Fellowship (NMF) awardees. NMF raises funds from foundations, corporations, and individual donors for the specific purpose of providing partial financial aid to all minority medical students enrolled in any U.S. school, provided the student requires financial aid. About 75 percent of minority students apply for this aid. Newsletters gave the names of all former NMF awardees. Unpublished NMF data provided information concerning all applicants whose family incomes made them ineligible for financial aid. Minority applicants who never applied to NMF could probably be assumed to be from families with higher incomes, as student affairs deans knew the income levels within which the minority students would be found ineligible to receive grants. In 1969 NMF made awards on the basis of need plus competitive scholastic merit; but from 1970 on, awards were made solely on the basis of need. Only Blacks received grants up to 1970. Therefore, we have data that describe the GME-1 program location decisions of minority interns with progressive degrees of economic disadvantage, and from all underrepresented groups, but not a complete sample.

A total of 2,109 minority students were identified and data obtained on their sex, year of graduation, medical school, ethnic membership, and NMF status. GME-1 hospital data were compiled on location of the hospital, its medical school affiliation, type of governance, percentage of foreign medical graduates on the house staff, and percentage of unfilled residency positions. A control group of 2,191 randomly chosen nonminority students were selected for the same 1973–77 period, and similar data were compiled for them. The control group was selected as follows: once a minority graduate was identified on the NIRMP alphabetical list, the next subsequent name was selected as a nonminority control. We did not use the name if it might possibly have been a minority applicant (Hispanic surname, or from a predominantly Black medical school). We would estimate that our nonminority sample probably inadvertently contains about twenty minority interns through this sampling method. We later dropped some interns from both groups because of incomplete data. Approximately two hundred nonminority interns were dropped from analysis of findings in this chapter because we observed that they were graduates of foreign medical schools.

The hospital data were obtained from the "Green Book," the *Directory of Accredited Residencies* (AMA 1976a), using 1975–76, which gave data on hospitals with which the 1974 graduates were matched, as a typical academic year.

For most of the printouts on which geographic location data were available, there were 1,982 students in the minority sample and 1,885 nonminorities in the control group. The minority group was further divided as follows: 1,666 Blacks, 204 Mexican Americans, 84 Mainland Puerto Ricans, 23 Native Americans, and 5 whose ethnicity was not specified.

From the AAMC data (AAMC 1978, 63), the 1,885 member nonminority control group represents a 3.1 percent sample of the 61,518 nonminority medical students who graduated from 1973 to 1977, while the 1,982 minority students represent a 45.3 percent sample of the 4,370 minority students who graduated during that period. This method was most successful in identifying 84 Mainland Puerto Ricans (49.4 percent of 170); 1,666 Blacks (48.5 percent of 3,437); 204 Mexican Americans (32.1 percent) of 635; and least successful in identifying 23 Native Americans (18 percent of 128). Minority graduates in those years represented 6.6 percent of all medical school graduates.

Our data do not include minority students who were not identified on the Med-Mar Register, those who did not apply to NMF, and those who did not use the NIRMP. A study of all U.S. graduates in 1976 (Cuca 1977, 164) found that 13,505 (98 percent) applied to NIRMP, of whom 89 percent (11,728) followed through. The others withdrew or failed to follow through with the match, at a rate of 10 percent of nonminorities and 20 percent for minorities. An additional 8 percent of all U.S. graduates failed to match. Therefore, assuming the same participating and matching rates found in the 1976 AAMC study, 1,885 nonminorities represent a 3.67 percent sample of all 50,938 nonminority participants who matched. The 1,983 minorities are only a little over 60 percent of the 3,000 or so minority NIRMP participants who matched. By these estimates, minorities represented 5.8 percent of all NIRMP applicants. We believe both our minority and nonminority samples are sufficiently large and representative to indicate valid trends.

Given that the data on our minority sample do not include the 30 percent of minority graduates who fail to use the NIRMP (2 percent never apply, another 20 percent withdraw from the match to make their own arrangements, and another 8 percent fail to match), we could have obtained no more than 70 percent of all minority graduates.

While it is commonly supposed that most minority students who apply to medical school willingly designate themselves as such, believing it to be to their advantage to do so, this assumption had not been subjected to adequate study. Dr. Valerie Miké, chief statistical consultant to the first part of this study, suggested examination of that issue. The obvious question was whether those minority interns who failed to indicate their minority group status did so because they did not wish to associate with minority people or to be identified with them, or because they were fearful that knowledge of their race would be used against them in some way by Whites? Both of these possible attitudes would influence their internship choices, but in different directions. Furthermore, what can we learn about the internship choices of minority graduates who do not use the NIRMP?

Examining 1976 data more intensively, I looked at those medical schools at the top of the list that contributed 200 of the 615 minority interns in our sample for that year. From a variety of data sources I put together as much information as I could gather concerning the internship choices of all minority students graduating from those schools in 1976 (J. Hodge-Jones, personal communication; W. Jordan, personal communication; both Hodge-Jones and Jordan have compiled questionnaire data on residency choices of minority students). My efforts to clarify these issues were diligent, but they cannot be considered definitive.

In general Howard and Meharry graduates were believed not to participate in the NIRMP as often as those from other schools because their historical exclusion from most postgraduate training led graduates from these schools to apply for internships in teaching hospitals associated with their own Black schools, or to the small number of hospitals known to accept Blacks. In 1976, our review of all data showed that Howard graduated eighty-six minority students, of whom only forty-eight used NIRMP; Meharry graduated eighty-seven, of whom only forty-three used NIRMP. This yielded a combined Howard and Meharry NIRMP participation rate of only 52.6 percent. Looking at the hospitals selected by those who did not participate in NIRMP clearly indicated that they were associated with their medical schools, or they were associated with a city, county, or the federal government; all these hospitals served predominantly Black patient populations.

Another nine medical schools contributed the next largest proportions of our minority intern sample during the study period. In 1976 alone, these schools contributed the following numbers of minority graduates: College of Medicine and Dentistry of New Jersey (27); University of Illinois (Chicago) (24); UC San Francisco (23); SUNY Buffalo (21); Harvard (19); UCLA (16); Case Western Reserve University (16); University of Michigan (15); and Columbia Physicians and Surgeons (12). Of the 163 minority students they graduated, 156 (95.7 percent) participated in the NIRMP. Those who did not participate came from the following schools: SUNY Buffalo (10), UC San Francisco (5), College of Medicine and Dentistry of New Jersey (5); University of Illinois (3); Case Western Reserve (2) and the University of Michigan and UCLA (1 each). Again, the twenty-seven who did not participate went mainly to hospitals that were closely associated with their medical schools or to hospitals under city, county or other government auspices. Those hospitals usually were not highly competitive and had high proportions of foreign medical house staff and many unfilled positions. This suggested that minority students who graduated from these schools who did not use the NIRMP were academically below average, as is generally found to be true of nonminority students who do not use the NIRMP.

This generalization probably does not hold true for Howard and Meharry graduates. No obviously different pattern of specialty choice appeared, either in the twenty-seven non-NIRMP participants from the nine schools or the larger number of eighty-two from Howard and Meharry. The overall NIRMP participation rate for these top eleven schools in 1976 was 73.5 percent. Howard and Meharry, with their low participation rates, pulled down the aggregate rate for the top eleven schools. However, since those two schools contributed only 13 percent of our original 1976 sample, it is apparent that the minority participation rate for all medical schools would probably be close to the 80 percent that had been reported in the AAMC study of all 1976 graduates mentioned earlier (Cuca 1977).

Examining the same top eleven medical schools for 1976, we found that 200 of our sample of 615 had come from those schools, had been located by us, and were in our sample. We had not found an additional 31 who had used NIRMP. Five of those, from four different schools, were missed through lack of diligent search, as we should have found them by our method. However, 26 of the 31 had neither indicated their minority status on Med-Mar, nor had applied to NMF for financial aid. Those minority NIRMP candidates who had not designated their minority status again came in large numbers from the predominantly Black medical schools in 1976. Numerically they were found as follows: Meharry (6), Howard (4), University of Michigan (4), SUNY (Buffalo) (3), UC San Francisco (5), University of Illinois (2), Columbia Physicians and Surgeons (1). However, none were found at UCLA, Harvard, or the College of Medicine and Dentistry of New Jersey.

Since the group consisted of only 26 individuals, it is difficult to generalize. Our superficial examination of the hospitals or of the specialty training programs selected by these interns turned up no obvious differences between them and their minority classmates. However, these students probably were better off financially than others, as may be assumed from their not having applied to NMF for aid. While it is undoubtedly true that minority physicians would and should respond to the economic opportunities and other social advantages that influence all other physicians, their location decisions have been seriously constrained by past and current racial and ethnic discrimination that specifically delimits their opportunities for housing, jobs, incomes, education, and civil rights within a given state or region.

In summary, comparisons are made between the GME-1 training program choices of a sample of 2,109 minority graduates and 2,121 randomly selected nonminority graduates excluding about 200 foreign medical graduates in the nonminority group, all of whom had been alphabetically listed as having used the NIRMP in 1973, 1974, 1975, 1976, and 1977. Since the NIRMP data did not provide minority group identification, our most difficult task was that of ascertaining their minority group membership from the following additional sources: the minority premedical student registry (MED-MAR), provided by the AAMC Office of Minority Affairs, which sends the names of minority students applying to medical schools to all of the schools; and newsletters and other income status information from National Medical Fellowships.

Data on specialty choice was obtained on a total of 2,092 minority and 2,114 nonminority medical school graduates in the period 1973–77. Sample sizes for given years reflected the number of identifiable minority graduates admitted to medical school and therefore were unequal in the various years. In general, students who graduated in 1973 began medical school in 1969, four years earlier. Most of the minority sample was Black. Table 11 gives an idea of the serial composition of our total sample. Clearly Blacks were the dominant group. Aggregate numbers of other underrepresented minorities for the five-year period were Mexican Americans, 233, Mainland Puerto Ricans, eighty-five, and Native Americans, twenty-nine. A few students from both samples were dropped from the computer printouts because of coding errors or incomplete data.

TABLE 11. **Serial Composition of the Sample**

Year	Nonminorities		Blacks
1973	166		165
1974	306		276
1975	486		402
1976	588		466
1977	568		436
Total	2,114		1,745
		Other minorities	347
		Total	2,092

PROBLEM

The purpose of the study reported here was to determine if differences exist in trends of geographic location and specialty choice between minority and nonminority physicians in their Graduate Medical Education Year 1 (GME-1) training programs. Choice of specialty training will be discussed in the next chapter. I assumed that location of training programs was even more important than location of the medical school in determining where the physician would later decide to practice, although those factors are usually linked. The study concentrated primarily on the distribution differences of all minority groups combined, even though Blacks greatly outnumbered all other minorities in the sample. Wherever possible, data have been analyzed by the various subdistribution groups of Mexican Americans, Mainland Puerto Ricans, and Native Americans. In the past, studies of this kind were thwarted by lack of reported data on the ethnicity of medical students or physicians, as well as by the fact that all minorities combined were previously so small a number. The AAMC does not release information on the ethnic identification of individuals graduating from medical schools.

RESULTS

PRODUCTION OF INTERNS BY STATE OF ORIGIN

In 1972, the National Medical Association Foundation, an organization of Black physicians, surveyed by mail all fifty-eight hundred known Black physicians in the United States. The response rate was 60 percent (Crocker 1975). The study replicated Haynes's finding (Haynes 1969) that the states in which Black physicians are trained reflects the dominance of Howard and Meharry: District of Columbia (because Howard is located there) educated 44 percent; Tennessee (because of Meharry's location) 39 percent; Michigan (University of Michigan and Wayne State University) about 4.5 percent; Ohio (Ohio State and Case Western Reserve) 3.0 percent; Illinois (University of Illinois) 2.0 percent; and all other states contributed the remaining 6.5 percent. Historically, Howard and Meharry have been national resources for Black medical students. For example, in 1977, only 13 percent of Howard's students came from the District of Columbia, and only 16 percent of Meharry's students came from Tennessee (AAMC 1977, table 2-B). The vast majority of nonminority medical students, on the other hand, usually attend public or private medical schools within their own region or within their state of residence.

Table 12 shows the top ten states in rate of production of medical graduates, or interns. We can note the close similarity, and therefore the representativeness, of our nonminority sample of 1,885 for the 1973–77 period as compared to the total sample of 11,401 interns for the year 1976. We used 1976 because it included almost all the interns or GME-1 placements for that year, although it does not include those who went directly into GME-2 programs (AMA 1977, 20). It also can be seen that in general the top ten states produced just over half of all the medical school graduates.

Looking at our minority sample, we see that Tennessee (because Meharry is located in Nashville) and the District of Columbia (where Howard is located) occupy much higher ranks than they do in the nonminority sample, where the District of Columbia ranks thirteenth and Tennessee twelfth. The top ten states in minority intern production are responsible for turning out a greater percentage (76.6 percent) of all minority graduates than do the top ten states for nonminority graduates (only 57.9 percent).

While they contained half the Black population (53 percent according to the 1970 census), the southern states produced comparatively few minority graduates, calling attention to the continuing inequity of human services and economic parity in that part of the country. Table 13 compares the production of minority and nonminority graduates from the ten states with the highest percentage of Black population. States in the Deep South regularly generated lower-than-expected percentages of minority graduates.

The popularity of a given medical school reflects the mutual choice of both the applicant and the school for each other. A simple listing of the

TABLE 12. Top Ten States in Production of Interns

Rank	All 1976 Interns (N = 11,401)			1973–77 Nonminority Sample (N = 1,885)			1973–77 Minority Sample (N = 1,982)		
1.	New York	1,307	11.5%	New York	194	10.3%	New York	273	13.8%
2.	Pennsylvania	908	8.0%	Pennsylvania	155	8.2%	California	232	11.7%
3.	Illinois	800	7.0%	Illinois	147	7.8%	Tennessee	158	8.0%
4.	California	730	6.4%	Texas	111	5.9%	Pennsylvania	152	7.7%
5.	Texas	633	5.6%	California	109	5.8%	District of Columbia	149	7.5%
6.	Ohio	494	4.3%	Ohio	96	5.1%	Massachusetts	139	7.0%
7.	Michigan	467	4.1%	Michigan	77	4.1%	Michigan	126	6.4%
8.	District of Columbia	401	3.5%	Massachusetts	71	3.8%	Illinois	123	6.2%
9.	Massachusetts	391	3.4%	North Carolina	70	3.7%	Texas	85	4.3%
10.	Missouri	322	2.8%	Missouri	60	3.2%	Ohio	81	4.1%
	Total	6,453	56.6%		1,090	57.9%		1,518	76.7%

Source: Figures for all 1976 interns from Directory of Accredited Residencies (1977).

top twenty-five choices of medical school for both minority and nonminority medical school graduates reemphasizes some of the points already made (see table 14). For example, the top twenty-five schools graduated 56.1 percent of all the minority sample, but the top twenty-five schools for the more widely dispersed nonminority sample graduated only 36.9 percent of that group. Only eight of the top twenty-five choices were shared by both minority and nonminority graduates. While the Ivy League schools and the high-prestige private and state universities generally dramatically opened up to minority students, the same cannot be said for the large state universities either in the South or the Midwest.

STATE GME-1 RETENTION RATES

Not a single state is spared some manifestation of severe physician shortage somewhere within its boundaries. A given state must maximize efforts to attract or retain at least as many interns as it produces, whether they are produced from within the state's own boundaries or outside, in order to maintain if not improve its physician-to-population ratio. While an increase in the number of physicians alone might not solve all of those shortage problems that result primarily from maldistribution, it is almost certain that reduction in the total number of physicians would hamper future resolution efforts.

Table 15 presents an analysis of the net gain or loss of interns for selected states, comparing the flow of minority and nonminority interns

TABLE 13. Production of Interns in Ten States with Highest Proportion of Black Population

State	Black Population %	Percentage of Nationwide Minority Sample Produced ($N = 1,982$)	Percentage of Nationwide Nonminority Sample Produced ($N = 1,885$)
District of Columbia	71.1	7.5	2.6
Mississippi	36.8	0.5	1.8
South Carolina	30.5	0.5	1.2
Louisiana	29.8	1.5	2.9
Alabama	26.2	0.9	1.3
Georgia	25.9	1.0	2.7
North Carolina	22.2	2.2	3.7
Virginia	18.5	0.9	3.2
Arkansas	18.3	0.8	1.4
Maryland	17.8	2.5	2.0

Note: Figures on Black population of states are from 1970 U.S. Census data. Interns are 1973–77 graduates from U.S. medical schools.

within a given state. These data do not apply to specific individuals, but rather to the sum total of all medical students graduated from all schools within a state, and the sum total of all interns, from any school in any state, choosing a GME-1 program located within that same state.

Table 15 can be read as follows: New York had 350 minority interns from our sample in the 1973–77 time period, while it graduated only 273, showing a net gain of 4.7 percentage points (350 being 17.7 percent of the interns and 273 representing 13.0 percent of graduates). Compared with nonminorities in the same time period, 198 were interns in the state, while 194 medical school graduates were produced, a gain of only 1.3 percentage points. The observed difference in gain of minorities compared to non-minority interns was statistically significant (calculating the significance of

TABLE 14. Medical Schools Preferred by Minority and Nonminority Samples

	Minority Sample (%)		Nonminority Sample (%)
1. Meharry	7.0	1. Indiana	2.7
2. Howard	5.5	2. Ohio	1.9
3. Harvard*	3.6	3. Wayne*	1.8
4. University of Michigan*	3.3	4. Nebraska	1.7
5. UC San Francisco	3.1	5. Baylor*	1.7
6. Columbia (P.&S.)*	2.7	6. Tennessee	1.7
7. Illinois (Chicago)*	2.4	7. Texas (Galveston)	1.7
8. SUNY (Buffalo)	2.1	8. Harvard*	1.6
9. UCLA*	2.0	9. Illinois (Chicago)*	1.6
10. Case Western Reserve	1.9	10. Mississippi	1.6
11. New Jersey C.M.D.*	1.9	11. Jefferson	1.5
12. Wayne*	1.9	12. University of Michigan	1.5
13. Cornell	1.7	13. Virginia Medical College	1.5
14. Yale	1.7	14. Hahnemann	1.4
15. U. of Southern California	1.6	15. Iowa	1.4
16. Temple	1.6	16. Texas (Southwestern)	1.4
17. Tufts	1.6	17. Georgia	1.4
18. University of Pennsylvania	1.5	18. Oklahoma	1.3
19. Baylor*	1.4	19. St. Louis	1.3
20. Stanford	1.3	20. New Jersey C.M.D.*	1.3
21. Johns Hopkins	1.3	21. Arkansas	1.3
22. SUNY (NYC)	1.3	22. Cincinnati	1.3
23. Pittsburgh	1.3	23. New York Medical College	1.3
24. New Mexico	1.2	24. UCLA*	1.2
25. New York University	1.2	25. Columbia (P.&S.)*	1.2
Total	56.1		36.9

*School appears on both lists

TABLE 15. Net Gain or Loss of Interns in Selected States, 1973–77

	Minority			Nonminority			Significantly Different Percent Change
	Interns (N = 1,982)	Graduates (N = 2,099)	Percentage Point Gain	Interns (N = 1,885)	Graduates (N = 2,090)	Percentage Point Gain	
1. New York	350	273	4.7	198	194	1.3	**
2. California	338	232	6.0	189	109	4.8	**
3. Illinois	147	123	1.5	68	147	-2.4	**
4. Michigan	136	126	0.9	92	77	1.2	
5. Texas	115	85	1.8	144	111	2.3	
6. Ohio	104	81	1.3	87	96	0.0	*
7. Pennsylvania	97	152	-2.3	120	155	-1.0	
8. Maryland	70	49	1.2	34	37	0.0	
9. Georgia	61	21	2.1	48	50	0.1	**
10. District of Columbia	59	149	-4.2	20	50	-1.2	**
11. Massachusetts	57	139	-3.7	79	71	0.8	**
12. Missouri	41	50	-0.3	66	60	0.6	
13. New Jersey	40	53	-0.5	24	35	-0.4	
14. Louisiana	36	29	0.4	31	54	-0.9	
15. Indiana	33	25	0.5	39	57	-0.6	
16. Florida	32	25	1.2	53	41	0.8	
17. Connecticut	29	39	-0.4	44	21	1.3	**
18. Colorado	27	17	0.6	33	22	0.6	
19. Arizona	27	7	1.1	30	14	0.9	
20. North Carolina	26	43	-0.7	76	70	0.7	
21. Virginia	22	19	0.2	44	60	-0.6	
22. Mississippi	12	9	0.2	17	33	-0.7	
23. Alabama	9	18	-0.4	17	24	-0.2	
24. Arkansas	6	15	-0.4	15	27	-0.5	
25. Tennessee	5	158	-7.3	32	54	-0.9	**
26. New Mexico	5	26	-1.0	4	7	-0.1	
27. South Carolina	5	8	-0.2	12	23	-0.5	
28. All other states	93	128	-0.2	269	391		

*p < .05.   **p < .01.

differences in percentage of change between the two groups). As can be seen in table 15, New York, California, and especially Illinois (among the top three states in number of minority interns produced) all show highly significant differences in rate of gain for minority physicians in training. While both minority and nonminority interns flocked to California, the migration was relatively less pronounced among minority graduates. Minority interns favored Illinois during the same period that nonminority interns were strongly avoiding the state. While both minority and nonminority interns favored New York, the minority preference was much greater.

The inflow and outflow suggest that the Midwest states with large urban Black populations (Illinois, Michigan, Ohio, Indiana) were all gaining minority physician trainees, while nonminority interns showed a gain only in Michigan. The same general trend is suggested for several southern states with large urban Black populations (Georgia, Louisiana, and Maryland).

The low retention rates for Blacks in the District of Columbia and in Tennessee are explained because the many Blacks graduating from the predominantly Black medical schools located in those states far exceeded the postgraduate training positions and subsequent practice opportunities offered in those two states. Other southern states, especially those with large Black rural populations, attracted few Black interns. Other states in the North with relatively small Black populations, but with high-prestige medical schools where relatively more Blacks then received their medical education (Pennsylvania, Massachusetts, Connecticut), would probably continue to produce more minority graduates than they could utilize.

VARIATIONS IN GME-1 LOCATION AMONG MINORITY SUBGROUPS

The addition of as few as twenty new minority physicians in almost any state would favorably improve access to physicians care by the minority population of that state, whereas the same number of new nonminority physicians would have much less effect.

Table 16 shows the geographic distribution of GME-1 placements for the various minority subgroups. There it can be seen that Black interns, like the Black population, were concentrated in large cities to a greater extent than is true of the whole population. Each of the top ten states have major cities with high percentages of Black people. The highly segregated neighborhoods in which most Blacks in these large cities live are almost like separate cities. According to the 1970 census, the top ten states, in

total Black population, were New York, Illinois, California, Texas, Georgia, North Carolina, Louisiana, Florida, Pennsylvania, and Michigan
(U.S. Dept. of Commerce 1976, 1–48). With the exception of Pennsylvania and North Carolina, Black GME-1 interns were attracted to those
states at rates that exceeded those of Black graduates produced. This definitely suggests a probable improvement in potential physician services for
the Black populations in those states. It occurred even though, as can be
seen in table 15, southern states were simultaneously losing nonminority
interns.

Table 16 also shows that the small subgroup of Mexican American interns went to states where their population is clustered, such as California
and Texas, as well as other southwestern states. (The top ten states in Mexican American population were California, Texas, Utah, Illinois, New
Mexico, Colorado, Michigan, Washington, Kansas, and Florida [U.S.
Dept. of Commerce 1973].)

Similarly, Native Americans were drawn to states where they lived.
Their top ten states in population were Oklahoma, Arizona, California,
New Mexico, North Carolina, Washington, South Dakota, New York,
Montana, and Minnesota. Mainland Puerto Ricans tend to cluster in
New York City, other large cities in the East, and in Puerto Rico. The top
ten states in Puerto Rican population were New York, New Jersey, California, Illinois, Pennsylvania, Connecticut, Florida, Massachusetts, Ohio,
and Indiana (U.S. Dept. of Commerce 1976, 1–48). GME-1 locations,
therefore, indicate that these minority subgroups were migrating in a
population pattern characteristic of others of their ethnic origin and
identity group.

TABLE 16. GME-1 Placements by Minority Subgroup, Top Ten States

Black (N = 1,666)		Mexican American (N = 204)		Mainland Puerto Rican (N = 84)		Native American (N = 23)	
New York	18.4%	California	37.3%	New York	41.7%	California	13.0%
California	15.0%	Texas	26.5%	California	8.3%	Michigan	13.0%
Illinois	8.5%	Arizona	6.9%	Pennsylvania	7.1%	Pennsylvania	8.7%
Michigan	7.7%	Colorado	4.4%	Puerto Rico	6.0%	Colorado	8.7%
Ohio	6.2%	New York	2.5%	New Jersey	4.8%	New York	4.3%
Pennsylvania	5.2%	Illinois	2.5%	Massachusetts	3.6%	Arizona	4.3%
Maryland	3.8%	Utah	2.5%	Maryland	3.6%	Maryland	4.3%
Texas	3.5%	New Mexico	2.5%	Michigan	2.4%	New Jersey	4.3%
Georgia	3.5%	Indiana	2.0%	Texas	2.4%	Washington	4.3%
District of Columbia	3.4%	Michigan	1.5%	Arizona	2.4%	Oklahoma	4.3%
Total	75.2%		88.6%		82.3%		69.2%

GME-1 PLACEMENTS OF MINORITY INTERNS BY ECONOMIC DISADVANTAGE

We identified three subclassifications of the combined minority sample according to degrees of economic disadvantage, and our relevant findings appear in table 17. Our assumption is that from 1973 to 1977, National Medical Fellowship grant recipients ($N = 1,388$) were from families with the lowest incomes. The actual average family income was $8,880 for 1,190 families with reported income; there were 324 with no reported income. Next, we assumed that those who applied for but did not receive NMF grants ($N = 277$) had higher family incomes. (Their actual average family income was $14,960 for 227 families with reported income; 50 reported no family income.) Our next assumption was that those who never had applied for an NMF grant probably came from families with still higher family incomes, and of those there were 317 whose average family income could of course not be calculated.

Table 17 shows the top ten states preferred by the lowest of these economic subgroups, ranked in terms of numbers and percentages of minority interns who located there, with the comparable figures for the other two subgroups for those states. We found a statistically significant similarity of geographical distribution, comparing those who received NMF grants with those whose requests were rejected (the Kendall rank correlation was .64, which is significant at almost the $p = .01$ level) and also on comparison with those who never applied for an NMF grant (Kendall rank correlation is .75, significant at the $p = .01$ level). In other words,

TABLE 17. Placement of Minority Interns, by Economic Subgroup

NMF Grant Request Accepted ($N = 1,388$)				NMF Grant Request Rejected ($N = 277$)				NMF Grant Request Never Made ($N = 317$)			
State	Rank	N	%	State	Rank	N	%	State	Rank	N	%
New York	1	244	17.6	New York	1	54	19.5	New York	1	52	16.7
California	2	238	17.1	California	2	52	18.8	California	2	48	15.1
Illinois	3	111	8.0	Illinois	7	14	5.1	Illinois	3	22	6.9
Michigan	4	102	7.3	Michigan	6	15	5.4	Michigan	6	19	6.0
Texas	5	79	5.7	Texas	4	17	6.1	Texas	4	19	6.0
Ohio	6	73	5.3	Ohio	3	19	6.9	Ohio	8	12	3.8
Pennsylvania	7	63	4.5	Pennsylvania	5	15	5.4	Pennsylvania	5	19	6.0
Georgia	8	46	3.3	Georgia	9	11	4.0	Georgia	20	4	1.3
Maryland	9	44	3.2	Maryland	11	7	2.5	Maryland	7	19	6.0
Massachusetts	10	42	3.0	Massachusetts	10	8	2.9	Massachusetts	13	7	2.2
Total		1,042	75.0			212	76.6			221	70.0

there are no significant geographical GME-I location differences between economically disadvantaged minority interns with more economically advantaged minority interns as we defined them, even though average family incomes for these two subgroups were as wide apart as nine thousand and fifteen thousand dollars.

One possible interpretation of this finding is that income levels are not significant within that range of difference, given the other similarities between these subgroups of highly educated minority students. Another possible interpretation is that the more economically advantaged subgroups are not large enough to establish separate opinion and behavior trends. And there is also the opinion that minority group identification by itself has greater influence than income on choice of intern location, at least within the minority sample of interns taken as a whole. Data on income stratification and GME-I location choices within the minority intern sample are insufficient because the number of members of the other ethnic subgroups is so small. For Blacks, whose numbers are predominant in each income subgroup, ethnicity almost certainly is stronger than income level in influencing their GME-I location decisions, considering the history of racial segregation already reviewed.

DISCUSSION

IMPLICATION OF MINORITY MEDICAL SCHOOL GRADUATION TRENDS

In a concise report (DHEW 1978b, 31) on minority medical student programs, covering roughly the 1970–76 period, the DHEW Office of Health Resources Opportunity pointed out that minority enrollment success had reached a plateau or was threatened with a future decline. This was not only because the numbers of qualified minority applicants was not increasing significantly, and because the cost of medical education was increasing and becoming a greater barrier, but also because some medical schools had not made sincere efforts to increase their minority enrollment.

This lack of commitment is not so obvious for Native Americans, Mexican Americans, and Puerto Ricans, because they might be expected to attend schools mainly in states where they predominantly reside. However, with Blacks residing as they do in all parts of the United States, of all Blacks in medical school in 1970, 64 percent were attending schools in only seven states. By 1974, those same seven states (California, District of Columbia, Massachusetts, New York, Pennsylvania, Tennessee, and Michigan) still were absorbing 61 percent of all Black students. Looking at medical schools more specifically, in 1976, a total of 51 of 113 schools excluding Howard and Meharry, admitted ten or more first-year minority students; 21 schools admitted from six to ten, but 41 schools admitted five or fewer. Those 41 schools were located in all geographic regions, represented both public and private schools, were located in metropolitan areas and less-dense population areas, and were located in areas with both large and small minority populations. Some were located in cities where other medical schools had managed to find more than ten medical students to admit.

Our data concerning minority graduation trends logically portray a pattern similar to admission trends. The increase in the enrollment of minority students nationwide, from less than 3 percent in 1969 to a 9 percent range in 1976, brought to the nation's schools not only a group of students with different racial backgrounds, but students who were not traditional in other ways as well (DHEW 1978b, 15–17). Minority student family income and education levels were lower; the minority students, especially the Blacks, came from smaller colleges often with inadequate resources; a greater proportion of students tended to be women; more minority students were older and already married, and more had come from the inner city.

While some medical educators felt there were no data to support the assumption that minority physicians would be any more likely than their nonminority peers to practice in areas with a shortage of physicians, that same study of minority medical students (DHEW 1978b) summarized questionnaire data from the minority medical students association that indicated otherwise. That association, the Student National Medical Association, produced results that revealed that 74 percent of minority students planned to do their residency training in the inner city, compared to 7 percent who chose metropolitan suburban areas; 14 percent who chose small to medium cities; 3 percent rural areas. One of my earlier studies (Curtis 1975) found that minority students succeeded 90 percent of the time in obtaining their first, second, or third choice of residency training; and for that reason it should be possible to determine whether or not minority graduates would in fact act on their stated intentions.

Minority graduates indicated on the SNMA questionnaire that they generally planned to do their residency training in an inner city area (74.3 percent), and half of them (50.5 percent) indicated they would like to locate their permanent practices there as well. It is of further interest to note that of the minority medical students who responded to the questionnaire (response rate is not given), 85 percent were Black. Of all respondents, 43.4

percent had grown up in metropolitan inner city neighborhoods, and 68.0 percent had attended medical schools in inner city neighborhoods. Unfortunately, that study did not similarly poll a matched group of nonminority medical students, but observation suggests no such past, present, or future magnitude of association with the inner city.

Subsequent data from the study we are reporting here will more clearly document how these minority and nonminority interns actually made their choices in relation to the inner city. In an earlier book, I had suggested that future minority physicians would naturally have career aspirations similar to their White colleagues, but that the persistence of residentially segregated neighborhoods, both in the inner city and in the suburbs, would coerce most minority physicians to serve a predominantly minority community (Curtis 1971, 150–54). Nothing in the data we report in the present or subsequent chapters can really answer questions as to whether minority interns are making their career training choices out of altruistic free choice, habit or tradition, a feeling of psychological or social coercion, lack of information, or for other reasons. There can be no doubt, however, that the career pathways of minority and nonminority students differ in a predictable and dramatic manner, beginning the first postgraduate medical school year. Nor can there be doubt that these career choice differences carry important social consequences and benefits, especially for previously medically underserved minority communities. Some states are shouldering more, and others less, than their fair share of the costs and benefits of these newly graduating minority physicians.

MINORITY AND NONMINORITY PHYSICIAN TO POPULATION RATIOS

Thompson (1974) summarized the basic difficulties in the problem of estimating the shortage of Black physicians, compared to other physicians, pointing out that in 1972, there was one physician for every 649 people, but the ratio was one Black physician for every 4,298 Blacks. This represented a worsening ratio for Blacks inasmuch as in 1942, there had been one Black physician for every 3,377 Blacks. While it is true that more White physicians were willing to accept Black patients in 1972, and Black physicians were not as strictly limited to all-Black clienteles, the racially integrated medical market was still of very minor dimensions. It should be remembered that nearly all patients of most Black physicians were Black, and except rarely, nonminority physicians avoid practicing in predominantly Black geographic areas or neighborhoods.

An analysis of net gain or loss of minority and nonminority physicians over a five-year period, such as we have reported, tells more about the end-state of minority physician manpower rather than nonminority physician manpower in a given area, because the beginning physician manpower pools for the two groups in a given state are of such different sizes. For example, assuming that nationwide there were approximately 350,000 nonminority physicians, of whom 15 per 1,000 retire or die annually (DHEW 1974, 157), and about 9,500 had graduated annually, only a 10 percent overall increase in physician manpower would have been achieved at the end of five years. On the contrary, with fewer than 6,000 Black physicians in 1973, at the beginning of the five-year period, assuming a similar retirement and death rate, and with 700 annual graduates over that time period, Black physician manpower increased by about 50 percent. The increased supply of other underrepresented minority groups was of even greater importance in terms of their small numbers at the outset.

Table 15 also shows that throughout our 1973–77 review period, nonminority interns tended to be leaving the South and even the Northeast. Despite this migration, the northeast region of the country continued to be relatively well supplied with nonminority physicians, using as a measure the number of states with more than 140 physicians per 100,000 population (Roback 1975). Many of these eastern states, like New York and New Jersey, were forced to rely heavily on foreign medical graduates to meet their physician manpower needs and demand, while the West Coast region is richly supplied with U.S. physicians. Serious physician shortages for nonminorities as well as others continued to be a problem in many of the relatively affluent midwestern states, as well as in the impoverished southern states.

This study confirmed the finding that Black physicians tend to migrate in the same pattern as the Black population at large. From findings reported here, we see the high percentage of our graduates moving to California or going to New York. But even in California, in 1972 there had been only one Black physician per 1,800 Black persons, in New York one per 3,000. In Washington, D.C., the best supplied of all, one Black physician per 1,100 (Thompson 1974) was still only about half the average American ratio. Thompson pointed out that this serious Black physician manpower shortage would only be corrected by the production of more Black graduates from all the nation's medical schools. In fact, we can see that with a total population of 22,500,000 Black Americans in 1970, it would have required 35,000 rather than 6,000 Black physicians to achieve parity with other Americans. Assuming present levels of minority medical school enrollment and retention, and further assuming similar rates of physician attrition, we can estimate that as of 1977 there were 9,000 U.S. Black physicians. With an estimated net yearly gain as great as 800, by 1987, there would be a total of 17,000 Black physicians, which still would be only half the 1970 ratio for the population as a whole.

SERVING PHYSICIAN SHORTAGE AREAS

It is sufficient reason to train more physicians from minority communities just because they deserve professional and educational opportunities equal to other Americans. One can reasonably neither expect nor require them to feel more obligated than other American physicians to serve the underserved. Moreover, as deVise (1973) has stated, the doctor-rich states like California will continue to attract larger numbers of medical graduates from states like Illinois, not only because of the appeal of California's climate and glamour, but also because it attracts several times more federal dollars than Illinois, for health care, health education, and health research. Each year, California educates only half as many doctors per capita as Illinois, but it receives twice as many interns, residents, and newly licensed physician practitioners.

We concur with deVise's suggestion that a more socially equitable result could be brought about by means of policy alterations in federal, state, and local financial incentives and sanctions, applicable to all physicians, and to all components of the health system. Our findings indicate, however, that even in the absence of a more soundly conceived general health policy, the recently enrolled minority interns were bringing about a more equitable redistribution of physician services. Our GME-1 trainees not only were receiving postgraduate training, but they also were the principal expert health care providers to many of the segregated communities to which they were migrating.

Koleda and Craig 1976 and Gray 1977 have discussed available data on the geographic distribution of Black physicians. While 53 percent of Blacks lived in the South, only 32 percent of active Black physicians resided there, and about twice as many Black physicians relative to Black population were located in the middle Atlantic and western states. However, 45 percent of Black interns and residents in 1973 were in the South, suggesting an increased inmigration of Black physicians. This preceded the graduation of significant numbers of the recently increased minority medical school enrollees. Like Gray, I doubt that so high a percentage would ultimately remain to practice in the South. For the entire 1973–77 period, southern states with large urban population centers, such as Maryland, Texas, Georgia, Louisiana, and Florida, showed net gains in minority interns. Blacks apparently would migrate to states in the industrialized South, but not to southern states with predominantly rural, uneducated, impoverished, and politically powerless Black populations. So long as the South had an average Black family income that was only 57 percent that of the White family, compared to 73 percent that of Whites in other regions, it was unlikely that Black physician migration could be sustained to the southern region as a whole.

Gray also noted that 92 percent of Black physicians, compared to only 76 percent of White physicians, lived in urbanized central city areas. I agree with her that recently graduated young physicians would continue to migrate to areas of greatest growth in Black population. In 1970, 70 percent of all Blacks, compared to only 59 percent of Americans generally, lived in such urban areas. It is my opinion, however, that urbanized Blacks were the only ones of their group who were educationally and financially able to seek out, demand, and use specialist physician services.

For the nonminority United States there is a close similarity between the regional distribution of total population, regional distribution of numbers of medical schools, of applicants to medical schools, and to numbers of graduates of medical schools, but not as close a correlation with regional location of hospitals selected for GME-1 residencies (Cuca 1977). For the minority U.S. community there was never as close a connection between population distribution and location of education and training opportunity. Only about a dozen hospitals would give an internship or residency appointment to a Black physician until just after World War II (Curtis 1971). Findings reported here indicate that the desegregation of medical education and of GME-1 training opportunities began to make an important contribution to a more equitable distribution of physician services to the whole American public. The general relegation of Blacks and other underrepresented minorities to a status of segregated and second-class citizenship constituted the fundamental constraint on the equalization of health services up until 1977. Improvements in fundamental civil rights will continue to improve the delivery of health and other human services.

CONCLUSION

A 70 percent sample of minority graduates from U.S. medical schools who matched through NIRMP (2,109 out of an estimated 3,061) were compared to a random sample of 2,121 nonminority graduates who also matched through NIRMP for the five-year period from 1973 to 1977, observing the geographic locations of their internship placements. The high-prestige private and public medical schools were producing relatively more minority graduates than many of the other large public medical schools in the nation. Comparing the net gain or loss of interns, states with large Black urban populations, whether in the North or South, seemed to attract and hold more Black interns, even when many of these same states were losing nonminority interns. The relatively smaller numbers of Mexican American, Mainland Puerto Rican, and Native American interns also seemed to be locating in states where their population groups predominantly lived. An analysis of GME-1 location choices revealed no differences between minority graduates whose family incomes were substantially lower than those who were better off financially. Affirmative action pressures in the form of incentives and sanctions should be exerted at the levels of individual medical schools, at state levels, at regional levels of the nation, and for the nation as a whole, to promote a more equitable increase in the numbers of young physicians from racially diverse backgrounds.

While there might be doubt concerning the existence of a genuine physician shortage for U.S. citizens as a whole, there is no doubt that a serious physician shortage for Blacks and for other underrepresented minority groups still existed in the mid-1970s. It was recommended that high and special priority be given to the need for further increases in their medical school enrollments. Minority medical school graduates such as the young physicians reported here already were beginning to equalize access to physician services for all Americans.

v. Comparing Specialty Choices

PROBLEM

IT WAS A MAJOR HOPE and expectation that the increased enrollment of minority students in U.S. medical schools would to some extent correct both the geographic and specialty maldistribution of physician manpower in this country. Specifically, federal health manpower, legislation, Public Law 94-484, provided financial aid incentives for newly graduated physicians to pursue careers in primary care medical specialties, and to locate in federally designated areas of physician shortage. Similar financial incentives also were directed at all medical center residency training programs, which were required to contribute increasing percentages of their trainees to the national pool of primary care physicians.

Historically, almost 85 percent of all minority physicians have graduated from the two predominantly Black medical schools, Howard and Meharry, having been excluded from other schools by a process either of de facto or de jure racial discrimination. It was not until after World War II that Blacks had any real opportunity to pursue postgraduate medical specialty training. In 1947 only 93 of the 4,000 known U.S. Black physicians were certified by any specialty board; by 1957, the number of specialists had risen to 320, and in 1969, 1,074 of the 6,000 Black physicians were board-certified specialists (Curtis 1971, 59). In 1973, only 22 percent of Meharry's 2,257 alumni and 26 percent of Howard's 2,756 alumni were board certified, while 43 percent of all American physicians held those credentials (Martin 1975). Minority physicians had received full specialty training at only about one-half the rate of other American physicians.

National, state, and local health care and health manpower policy and incentives should reflect the need to correct this historical disadvantage in medical education and training suffered by Blacks and other underrepresented ethnic minority groups. Specifically, minority group communities do indeed suffer from a shortage of primary care physicians, but they suffer from a still greater shortage of specialists in all fields as well. Public health policy, and health planning guidelines, should address both of these needs.

This demand and need will continue as long as the Black population continues to be concentrated in large urban centers, clustered in racially segregated neighborhoods, and there is a national commitment to provide all our citizens with a single high standard of medical, hospital, and health-related services.

As we have seen, a larger number of minority students than ever before have been graduating from the nation's schools, and entering postgraduate training programs. By 1980, we were in a position to answer two questions: (1) Are minority students now entering specialty training programs with the same frequency as their nonminority classmates? and (2) Are they choosing specialties in a similar or different pattern from that of their nonminority peers?

FINDINGS AND DISCUSSION

YEAR-TO-YEAR SPECIALTY CHOICE FREQUENCIES OF BLACK AND NONMINORITY INTERNS

Table 18 provides data on year-to-year specialty choices for Black and for nonminority interns in the major fields. Since Blacks made up the overwhelming proportions of all minority interns, their numbers are sufficiently large to make comment on meaningful year-to-year trends. Nonminorities are of course almost all White, and, therefore, this table provides the most direct comment on differences in specialty choice patterns between Black and White interns.

While flexible or rotating internships were chosen with roughly equal frequency by Blacks and Whites over the five-year period, the year-to-year trends add important information. The declining popularity of flexible programs was much more marked for nonminorities, dropping from 28 percent to about 7 percent, than for Blacks, who went from about 15 percent down to 10 percent.

General surgery programs were equally popular with both groups in the combined five-year period, and there was no clear pattern in the year-to-year trend.

Obstetrics and gynecology, on the other hand, was chosen by almost three times as many Black interns as by nonminorities, and year-to-year data suggest that this trend was sustained over the study period.

Internal medicine was chosen equally by Blacks and by nonminorities and was clearly the most frequently chosen of any specialty field. Family practice programs, however, were more popular with nonminority interns at times by a two to one margin, but the year to-year trend suggests that in the last year, Blacks were choosing this field with increasing frequency.

Pediatrics seems to have been slightly more popular with Black interns, but the year-to-year trend suggests that this field may be chosen equally by both groups.

Nonminorities seemed to choose all other fields with greater frequency. This category included all the other medical, surgical, and support specialty services.

COMPARING MALE AND FEMALE SPECIALTY CHOICES IN THE MINORITY AND NONMINORITY SAMPLES

Table 19 presents data on the entire minority sample, including all other ethnic underrepresented subgroups along with Blacks, compared with the

TABLE 18. Specialty Choices of Blacks and Nonminority Interns, 1973–77

Specialty	Total		1973		1974		1975		1976		1977	
	N	%	N	%	N	%	N	%	N	%	N	%
Flexible												
Black	215	12.3	25	15.2	52	18.8	49	12.2	45	9.7	44	10.1
Nonminority	280	13.2	47	28.0	75	24.5	55	11.3	61	10.4	42	7.4
Surgery												
Black	247	14.2	22	13.3	35	12.7	65	16.2	68	14.6	57	13.1
Nonminority	303	14.3	21	12.7	52	17.0	76	15.6	78	13.3	76	13.4
OB-GYN												
Black	207	11.9	16	9.7	29	10.5	47	11.7	54	11.6	61	14.0
Nonminority	94	4.4	4	2.4	9	2.9	25	5.1	25	4.3	31	5.5
Internal Medicine												
Black	600	34.4	62	37.6	90	32.6	144	35.8	160	34.3	144	33.0
Nonminority	718	34.0	47	28.3	96	31.4	179	36.8	201	34.2	195	34.3
Family Practice												
Black	130	7.4	9	5.5	8	2.9	28	7.0	41	8.8	44	10.1
Nonminority	257	12.2	13	7.8	23	7.5	59	12.1	91	15.5	71	12.5
Pediatrics												
Black	217	12.4	20	12.1	40	14.5	46	11.4	61	13.1	50	11.5
Nonminority	217	10.3	21	12.7	25	8.2	43	8.8	59	10.0	69	12.1
Other fields												
Black	129	7.4	11	6.7	22	8.0	23	5.7	37	7.9	36	8.3
Nonminority	245	11.6	13	7.8	26	8.5	49	10.1	73	12.4	84	14.8
Total												
Black	1,745	100.0	165	100.1	276	100.0	402	100.0	466	100.0	436	100.1
Nonminority	2,114	100.0	166	99.7	306	100.0	486	99.8	588	100.1	568	100.0

entire nonminority sample in the combined 1973–77 time period. The most immediately apparent observation is that there were more minority women in their total sample (23 percent) compared to nonminority women (only 16 percent), a difference that is statistically significant ($p <$ .01). We considered it important, therefore, to determine whether the men and women within these two samples were expressing different frequency patterns of specialty choice. We also had to observe the possibility that differences between the minority and nonminority samples as a whole might have come about just on the basis of a greater proportion of women within the minority sample, since it is a common observation

TABLE 19. **Minority and Nonminority Internships, by Sex and Specialty**

Specialty	Minorities			Nonminorities		
	% Choosing	N	% M/F	% Choosing	N	% M/F
Flexible	12.2			13.8		
Male		203	78.7		235	86.4
Female		55	21.3		37	13.6
Surgery	13.0			14.0		
Male		248	90.2		263	88.3
Female		27	9.8		35	11.7
Surgical specialty	2.2			3.0		
Male		39	84.8		54	84.4
Female		7	15.2		10	15.6
OB-GYN	10.4			4.2		
Male		163	74.4		69	77.5
Female		56	25.6		20	22.5
Internal Medicine	32.2			33.5		
Male		534	78.5		610	85.8
Female		146	21.5		101	14.2
Family Practice	9.3			11.3		
Male		152	77.2		215	85.7
Female		45	22.8		36	14.3
Pediatrics	12.2			9.8		
Male		143	55.6		153	73.9
Female		114	44.4		54	26.1
Psychiatry	3.2			4.0		
Male		52	76.5		66	77.6
Female		16	23.5		19	22.4
Others	5.1			6.7		
Male		87	79.8		118	31.9
Female		22	20.2		26	18.1
Total		2,109	100.0		2,121	100.0
Male		1,621	76.9		1,783	84.1
Female		488	23.1		338	15.9

that men and women physicians generally show different specialty career patterns.

FLEXIBLE PROGRAMS

No significant differences were observed between the percentages of minorities and nonminorities who chose flexible programs (12.2 percent versus 13.8 percent), nor in the relative proportions of men or women within either group who chose flexible programs (21.3 percent of minority women chose flexible programs compared to 13.6 of nonminority women, but these proportions were within the expected range of numbers based on the total number of women in each respective group).

SURGERY

Minority and nonminority interns chose GME-1 surgery programs with almost equal frequency (13.0 percent versus 14.0 percent). In the nonminority group, men preferred surgery significantly more frequently than women ($p < .05$), but the male preference for surgery programs was significantly greater among men in the minority group. Minority women chose surgery programs significantly less often ($p < .01$) compared to all others combined, and in separate comparisons to minority men, or nonminority men or women. While this is an interesting initial observation, we can only speculate that it may have been a result either of more vigorous recruiting of nonminority than of minority women in a response to affirmative action challenges, or that fewer minority women are interested in surgery.

OBSTETRICS AND GYNECOLOGY

Minorities chose programs in obstetrics and gynecology with significantly greater frequency than did nonminority classmates ($p < .01$). This preponderance of minority interns reflects the choice of women as much as men, since the sexes are represented in that specialty in the same proportions as in the overall minority sample. Among nonminority interns, women were more highly represented in this field than in the sample as a whole, but the finding is of only borderline statistical significance. A significantly greater proportion of minority women go into obstetrics and gynecology ($p < .01$).

MEDICINE

Minorities and nonminorities, as well as men and women within these groups, chose medicine programs in approximately proportionate numbers.

FAMILY PRACTICE

Significantly more nonminorities chose family practice ($p < .01$), but within both groups these programs were equally popular with men and women.

PEDIATRICS

Pediatrics was significantly preferred by minority interns over nonminorities ($p < .02$); and in both groups, there was a great overrepresentation of women ($p < .01$). Proportionately many more minority women ($p < .01$) entered this field. It is the strong popularity of pediatrics among minority women that accounts for its greater popularity with minority interns.

PRIMARY CARE GME-I PROGRAMS

Primary care programs are defined by NIRMP as consisting of internal medicine, family practice, and pediatrics; and the generalist specialties include obstetrics and gynecology and general practice (Graetinger 1978).

Defined in this way, minorities entered the generalist programs significantly more ($p < .01$) than nonminority interns; but there was no difference in their overall rates of entry into primary care programs as defined. In other words, the heavy participation of minorities in obstetrics and gynecology programs and the reclassification of that specialty from a specialty to a generalist category chiefly differentiate the specialty choice patterns of minority interns as more generalist in nature.

However, while there is no significant difference in the representation of men and women within the nonminority sample in terms of their participation in primary care or generalist programs, a significantly higher

TABLE 20. Specialty Choice Differences among Minorities, by Economic Status

	All Minorities (N = 2,016)		NMF Nonapplicant (N = 333)		NMF Reject (N = 274)		NMF Awardee (N = 1,404)	
	N	%	N	%	N	%	N	%
Flexible	260	12.9	40	12.0	40	14.6	180	12.8
Surgery	277	13.7	45	13.5	42	15.3	190	13.5
Surgical Specialty	47	2.3	10	3.0	5	1.8	32	2.3
Family Practice	198	9.8	34	10.2	27	9.8	137	9.7
Medicine	685	34.0	108	32.4	95	34.7	482	34.2
Psychiatry	68	3.4	12	3.6	7	2.6	49	3.5
OB-GYN	219	10.9	32	9.6	27	9.9	160	11.3
Pediatrics	262	13.0	52	15.6	31	11.3	174	12.7

proportion of minority women than their overall representation in the sample ($p < .01$) chose to go into the combined fields of internal medicine, family practice, and pediatrics, with or without combining these fields with obstetrics and gynecology.

We conclude that minority women more often chose programs in primary care or the generalist specialties ($p < .01$), and went into surgery programs less often compared to minority men, nonminority men, and nonminority women.

SPECIALTY CHOICE DIFFERENCES WITHIN THE MINORITY SAMPLE

ECONOMIC DISADVANTAGE WITHIN THE MINORITY SAMPLE

The data in table 20 show that minority group graduates did not make specialty choices in any demonstrable relationship to their financial circumstances. The assumptions we made about NMF in chapter 4 apply again here.

Clearly all the economic subgroups discussed in chapter 4 made similar specialty choices for their GME-1 year, a convincing demonstration that differences in financial resources, at least in the ranges described, exerted no measurable effect on the specialty training preferences of minority medical school graduates, even though the most economically disadvantaged group had average family incomes that were only slightly more than half that of the other groups.

ETHNIC MINORITY SUBGROUPS WITHIN THE MINORITY SAMPLE

Table 21 summarizes the GME-1 specialty choices for the four underrepresented minority subgroups: 1,745 Blacks, 233 Mexican Americans, eighty-five Puerto Ricans from the U.S. mainland, and twenty-nine Native Americans. Of course the latter two subgroups are so few in number that any trends are only suggestive.

Comparing Blacks to all the other minority groups combined revealed that significantly more of the other minority groups than Blacks went into family practice ($p < .01$). Except for Puerto Ricans, proportionately more Blacks went into internal medicine ($p < .01$). Their choices of surgery were not significantly different. However, the preference of minorities for obstetrics and gynecology reflects the choice of Blacks ($p < .01$) more than of the other minority subgroups. Also there was a suggestion of greater preference of Mexican Americans, compared to Blacks, for the support specialties (defined as pathology, anesthesiology, radiology, physical medicine, and diagnostic and therapeutic radiology [Graetinger 1978]), but this difference is not statistically significant.

DIFFERENCES WITHIN THE BLACK SUBGROUP

Table 22 shows differences within the Black subgroup. Our data revealed that Blacks who graduated from medical schools from 1973 to 1977 were not a homogeneous group. Take the most obvious first question: do graduates of Meharry choose different specialties than graduates of Howard? The answer is yes, there are significant differences. The pattern of specialty choices differs for Howard and for Meharry ($p < .01$; all Howard or Meharry graduates who were not Black excluded). A greater number of Meharry graduates went into flexible GME-1 programs; more Meharry interns went into surgery programs; fewer Meharry graduates went into internal medicine, the support specialties, and the medical or surgical specialties.

The overall pattern of specialty choice is different for Blacks who graduated from all other medical schools combined, compared either to Howard or to Meharry graduates. Table 22 shows that Howard graduates more closely resembled the graduates of predominantly White medical schools. Compared to Howard graduates, Blacks who graduated from predominantly White schools less often chose flexible programs, and more often chose medicine or family practice. Blacks in all categories show a

TABLE 21. Specialty Choice, by Minority Subgroup

	Black (N = 1,745)		Mexican American (N = 223)		Puerto Rican Mainland (N = 85)		Native American (N = 29)		Other Non-Black Minorities Combined (N = 337)	
	N	%	N	%	N	%	N	%	N	%
Flexible	215	12.3	33	14.7	8	9.3	4	13.8	45	13.3
Surgery	247	14.0	25	11.2	8	9.3	3	10.3	36	10.6
Surgical Specialty	26	1.5	3	1.2	0	0.0	2	6.9	5	1.5
OB-GYN	207	11.7	19	8.5	3	3.5	2	6.9	24	7.1
Pediatrics	217	12.4	31	13.8	17	19.8	3	10.3	51	15.1
Family Practice	131	7.4	47	21.0	10	11.6	8	27.6	65	19.2
Internal Medicine	600	34.1	44	19.7	35	40.7	6	20.6	85	25.2
Medical Specialty	61	3.5	7	3.0	2	2.3	1	3.4	10	2.9
Support Specialty	42	2.6	14	6.1	0	0.0	0	0.0	14	4.1

similar high frequency of choice of obstetrics and gynecology. More of Howard's graduates chose the support specialties, or medical or surgical subspecialties in comparison to other Black interns.

DISCUSSION

FLEXIBLE OR ROTATING INTERNSHIPS

Earlier we reported that these programs experienced a decline in popularity in the 1973–77 five-year period both for minority medical schools graduates (going from 15 to 10 percent) and even more for nonminority graduates (from 28 to 7 percent). This mirrors the finding reported by Graettinger (1978) on nationwide NIRMP trends that only about one-third as many U.S. graduates in 1974 went into flexible programs compared to U.S. graduates who entered flexible or rotating programs in 1977. Some six thousand of approximately seventeen thousand positions offered in all programs in 1974 were rotating or flexible, of which three thousand were filled; in 1977, of seventeen thousand positions offered, two thousand were flexible, and just a few over one thousand were filled (figures are rounded to the nearest thousand). Reasons for the declining popularity of these programs are complex, and have been reviewed by Graettinger (1978), but mainly reflect the increasing interest of U.S. graduates in pursuing some form of specialty training. At one time a broadly diversified or rotating postgraduate training, for one year after medical school graduation, was all that usually was required to apply for a license to practice medicine. This

TABLE 22. Specialty Choice within Black Subgroup, Historically Black Schools versus Others

	All Blacks (N = 1,745)		Schools other than Howard or Meharry (N = 1,473)		Howard and Meharry Combined (N = 272)		Meharry Alone (N − 149)		Howard Alone (N = 123)	
	N	%	N	%	N	%	N	%	N	%
Flexible	215	12.3	156	10.6	59	21.7	40	26.8	19	15.4
Surgery	247	14.0	207	14.0	40	14.7	30	20.1	10	8.1
Family practice	130	7.4	122	8.3	8	2.9	4	2.7	4	3.3
Internal medicine	600	34.1	543	36.8	57	21.0	23	15.4	34	27.6
OB-GYN	207	11.7	165	11.2	42	15.4	23	15.4	19	15.4
Pediatrics	217	12.4	189	12.8	28	10.3	15	10.1	13	10.6
All others	129	7.4	91	6.2	38	14.0	14	9.4	24	19.5

Note: The overall pattern of specialty choices of minority students at all other medical schools in comparison with minority students at either Howard or Meharry is statistically significant at $p < .01$. Howard and Meharry are also significantly different from each other ($p < .01$).

no longer is considered adequate. Further, several specialty boards abol-
ished the rotating or general internship as a required, separate, initial year
of training for certification in their field. The change in name as well as
purpose led to the decline in popularity of these programs.

In this light, it is important to note that Meharry graduates, unlike
other Blacks and other minority interns, were still selecting flexible or rotating internships more than twice as often as other minority interns. This
may mean that more Meharry graduates were planning to enter general
practice careers after a year of postgraduate training. Private communications with the dean's staff both at Meharry and at Howard indicated that
within the two years after 1977, increasing percentages of their graduates
were selecting primary care or other specialty programs, and fewer were
going into flexible programs.

ARE MINORITY STUDENTS ENTERING
SPECIALTY TRAINING AS FREQUENTLY AS
THEIR NONMINORITY CLASSMATES?
IF SO, SHOULD THEY?

Whether we consider the entire minority sample, as shown from data reported in table 19, or the Black subgroup only as shown in table 18, it
seems clear that minority graduates in the five-year 1973–77 time period
were beginning specialty training at a rate equal to that of their nonminority peers. This undoubtedly was the first five-year period in the history of
American medical education, or of American postgraduate medical training, for which this statement could be made. Undoubtedly, this was a notable achievement in the first decade of affirmative action minority admissions programs, which were undertaken with the aim of broadening and
diversifying the base of American medical manpower by removal of ethnic
barriers to medical educational opportunity.

Why is it a clear social and medical care gain that Blacks and other ethnic minorities should be specialized in equal proportions to their nonminority physician colleagues? Because even though only about 25 percent
of living Howard and Meharry alumni were board certified (compared to
43 percent of living alumni of other medical schools), this did not represent their free choice, but rather was the result of a century of racially discriminatory denial of training opportunity.

U.S. medical school graduates in the 1960s and 1970s became much
more completely specialized than ever before. Levit et al. (1974) tracked a
sample of graduates from the classes of 1960 and 1964 and found in 1974
that postgraduate education had become a standard component of an

American physician's education. In their sample of over thirteen hundred physicians, 90 percent had entered some form of residency training, 73 percent had completed their training, and about 62 percent had become board certified. It took at least twelve years after medical school graduation to obtain a reliable estimate of how many of them probably would eventually achieve board certification. Specialization will continue at this rate both for nonminority and minority physicians so long as it remains the only route to professional status, monetary reward, academic advancement, hospital admitting privileges, and inner feelings of personal achievement and self-esteem.

Most Black physicians, like their White colleagues, indicate that they limit their practice, or otherwise identify themselves as specialists, on the American Medical Association questionnaires periodically submitted to them. They do so whether they have passed their specialty board examinations and achieved formal certification status or not. While some physicians have completed all, and many have completed part, of their specialty training, equality of educational and training opportunity for minority physicians has only recently become a reality. Table 23 provides data on the self-designation of specialty practice as reported by alumni from all U.S. medical schools and from Howard and Meharry alumni. About one and a half times as many Black physicians were general practitioners in 1973 as all other physicians, certainly a significantly greater proportion of generalist or primary care physicians in that category alone. Surprisingly, however, it will be noted that the percentages of Blacks who identified themselves as specializing in the medical and surgical specialties rather closely match the percentages of nonminority practitioners so classifying themselves. A physician licensed to practice medicine within a given state

TABLE 23.   Self-Designated Specialty, Alumni of Historically Black Schools versus Others

	Alumni from all U.S. Schools (N = 286,741)		Howard Alumni (N = 2,756)		Meharry Alumni (N = 2,257)	
	N	%	N	%	N	%
General practice	45,471	15.6	609	22.1	620	27.4
Medical specialty	69,009	24.0	591	21.4	399	17.7
Surgical specialty	74,954	26.1	693	25.0	660	29.2
Other specialty	66,336	22.9	561	20.2	356	15.9
All others	30,971	10.9	302	10.8	222	9.7

Source: Data obtained from Martin 1975, 38,52, 53, 109.

is allowed freedom to practice as a generalist or as a specialist, with a great deal of local variation in standards of practice required. One can only conclude, therefore, that the aspiration level of all American physicians is highly similar, and that aspirations to high standards also are generally high, but that opportunity only now is at the point of converging these equal ambitions with equal skills. Many if not most Black patients, confined to segregated ghetto neighborhoods in large cities or in rural areas, were becoming the beneficiaries of more equal specialist health care.

At the same time, as the nation relaxes its racial restrictions and desegregates its living arrangements in all areas, Black and other minority physicians of the future will be prepared to join their nonminority peers in making equal leadership contributions to all areas of American medicine, not only as general practitioners but also as specialist consultants, teachers, researchers, administrators, and health planners and policymakers.

While we await the further desegregation of American society, including medical affairs, highly trained minority specialists will be required to operate first-class medical services in the hospitals, clinics, group practices, and private offices located in segregated neighborhoods. An argument therefore could be made for encouraging minority medical school graduates to enter specialty training programs, even in those specialties that currently are overcrowded with nonminority specialists. Without doubt this would increase the chances, within a city, county, or state, of having a specialist who would voluntarily choose, rather than be forced or required, to serve in an ethnically unpopular geographical area. Furthermore, it is degrading and demoralizing for Black Americans to live in a society in which all the experts and specialists are White.

ARE MINORITY INTERNS MORE LIKELY TO CHOOSE A PRIMARY CARE CAREER?

Minority women as a group stood out in the frequency with which they chose to go into the combined fields of family practice, medicine, and pediatrics, especially because of their high preference for pediatrics. In this they differed from minority males, as well as from nonminorities of either sex. Since women made up a relatively larger proportion of the minority sample, an increasing supply of minority interns will automatically increase the proportion of primary care interns. The proportionately greater number of minority women among minority medical students has been described by Johnson, Smith, and Tarnoff (1975) on students entering all U.S. medical schools in 1972–73: among Caucasians, 16 percent were female, among Blacks, 29 percent, Native Americans, 24 percent, Mexican Americans, 14 percent, and Puerto Ricans, 20 percent.

ARE MINORITY INTERNS MORE LIKELY TO ENTER ANY PARTICULAR SPECIALTY?

The answer is yes. Obstetrics and gynecology was preferred two to three times more often by Black medical school graduates, compared to other medical school graduates, and was chosen by Black men and women proportionately. One reason may be that the field is no longer generally popular with medical school graduates, does not attract the graduates with the highest academic records, and therefore is easier to enter with a good postgraduate training placement. This would not explain the fact that Blacks expressed the same decided preference for obstetrics and gynecology (Johnson, Smith, and Tarnoff 1975) at the time they applied to medical school. They also held on to their choice of this field with more than average tenacity compared to students who chose other fields, as was shown in a study of specialist choice stability, measuring specialty choice at the beginning and again at the end of the medical school years. That study (Cuca 1977) of all 1976 graduates of U.S. medical schools also found that Blacks more often selected public health, but in our sample so few students selected that field that we could not confirm that finding.

My speculation on the reasons for the popularity of obstetrics and gynecology are as follows: Blacks are attracted to obstetrics and gynecology because in earlier decades this specialty above all others was plagued by blatant racial prejudice and practice. Black women in past decades were not admitted to most women's hospitals in this country, even if they were attended by a White physician. Black medical students or practicing physicians usually were not allowed to examine or treat women patients except in racially segregated hospitals. This created an early, strong, and separate market demand for Black physicians to provide this special medical care for their Black women patients.

Blacks have been sensitive to the knowledge that their rates of maternal and infant mortality are higher than for the nonminority group, reflecting inequities in the general health care delivery and health maintenance systems.

Blacks have had higher than average rates of fertility, a larger family size, more out-of-wedlock, teenage, or other problem pregnancies. This has served to expose many young minority physicians to traumatic memories from personal family, and neighborhood experience, alerting them to special needs in this area. Problems dealing with sexually transmitted diseases, disorders of sexual function, and problems of infertility were also common, further explaining a stronger than usual demand for medical service in this area.

Obstetrics and gynecology had, for all the above reasons, been an especially necessary and popular field for many decades, and this factor of itself served as a magnet to attract more than an average number of young physicians into the field. Several of the great teachers on the faculty of Howard and at Meharry were specialists in obstetrics and gynecology (personal communications with deans). For example, among Howard's 2,756 alumni, an unusually large number of 266 (9.1 percent) identified themselves as obstetricians and gynecologists in 1973, second only to the 333 who identified themselves as internists; while for all 286,741 U.S. medical school alumni only 16,330 (or 5.6 percent) were in obstetrics and gynecology (Martin 1975).

Obstetrics and gynecology probably will attract and should continue to attract a greater than average proportion of minority physicians as long as the factors mentioned above continue to operate. It is a matter of social importance that physicians meeting these intimate and special needs receive the highest level of specialist training and skill. This is a good example of the desirability and fairness of setting different and higher objectives for allocations of training, and of other health services, in order equitably to meet a currently different level of health care need in a defined minority group community.

At the same time, it is clear that as the economic, social, and cultural life experiences of the various minority groups more closely approximate those of other Americans, their health needs and health-planning profiles will become increasingly similar to those of the nation at large. Recent gains made in postgraduate training opportunities for minority groups mean that we are putting an end to producing first-class and second-class physicians for first-class and second-class racial groups. Future American physicians will clearly be able to provide a single high level of sensitive health care and health maintenance for all patients who seek their services, and an increasingly well educated American public will eventually outgrow its preference for a racially segregated medical market.

SUMMARY

A sample of 2,109 minority graduates from U.S. medical schools were compared to a sample of 2,121 nonminority graduates for the five-year period 1973–77, comparing the internship programs for which they were matched through the National Intern and Resident Matching Program. While currently living Black physicians are board certified at only approximately half the rate of White physicians, recent minority medical school graduates are entering postgraduate specialty training programs in the same frequency as their nonminority peers. Some differences are noted: more minority interns select obstetrics and gynecology, fewer select family medicine programs. Minority women more often choose programs in pediatrics and less often choose programs in surgery, compared either to minority men or to nonminorities of either sex. Other findings suggest that important differences in specialty choice may be found within the minority group sample. Degree of economic disadvantage in family background of minority interns does not account for differences in specialty choice.

Health planning at national, state, and local regional levels should take into account the fact that minority communities, served predominantly by minority physicians, have been deprived of a fair share of specialists as well as general and primary health care practitioners. Equitable resource allocation should allow for increased numbers of minority physicians to be trained in all specialty areas, as these physicians will be the most likely resource for voluntarily directing and staffing the health and hospital facilities and programs to serve minority group communities.

VI. Affirmative Action

IN GRADUATE MEDICAL EDUCATION

EVEN MORE THAN undergraduate medical education, graduate medical education programs determine the future form and function of the national physician workforce. In recent decades, graduate medical education (GME) has come to rival and surpass the undergraduate system in complexity and size. While in 1940, just under six hundred hospitals offered a total of about five thousand residency training positions, in 1976, approximately seventeen hundred hospitals offered more than sixty-five thousand positions. In 1979 an AAMC survey of graduating students from U.S. schools showed that 93.2 percent intended to finish residency training to complete requirements for specialty certification (AAMC 1980, 115). Of students graduating in 1977, 87.5 percent entered residency training in a teaching hospital in which postgraduate training was provided by "full-time and voluntary members of medical school faculties" (25).

Candidates for graduate training programs are selected by the various clinical departments within a teaching hospital, rather than by an admissions committee representing the whole faculty. The competence of resident physicians who complete the training is determined by outside examiners of the specialty boards who specialize in that field. The training programs also are certified by outside specialists. However, despite this splintering of responsibility, the medical school faculties do in fact control more than 95 percent of all residency training positions through affiliation agreements. Indeed, in most major teaching hospitals, the same faculty member is the head of a given clinical department for both the hospital and the medical school. Even in situations of less close affiliation, the medical school department head will be responsible for the quality of the training program and its director.

Despite this medical faculty influence, there is a great deal of variation in quality of training from one special field to another within any teaching hospital. Severe shortages or surpluses of physicians from field to field necessarily lead to different recruitment and selection strategies. Serious current problems for GME to resolve, therefore, are those dealing with the necessity of improving consistency in quality of graduate training programs across the board, to coordinate training programs within a given institution, and to improve and secure future financial support for these important programs. Assuring equity of access to GME programs for all subgroups of our population has attracted less attention than the issue of admission to undergraduate medical schools. Problems of gaining access to graduate education programs within a given institution generally, but not always, follow the pattern of undergraduate medical school admission. In this chapter I present data on the major GME programs that are controlled by the medical schools.

PAST RACE PREJUDICE TOWARD BLACKS IN CLINICAL MEDICAL SETTINGS

Black students who attended predominantly White medical schools in earlier decades experienced great problems in their third and fourth clinical years when the time approached for them to go to the wards of the teaching hospital. Until the mid-1960s, Blacks in many parts of the nation had difficulty in gaining entrance to hospitals either as patients, nurses, medical students, residents, or staff physicians. Some of the predominantly White medical schools, with their small number of Black students, arranged in the 1920s and 1930s for these students to be transferred to Howard or Meharry for instruction in their last two clinical years. While this practice gradually had changed by the 1940s, it persisted well into the 1940s for Black students scheduled to do clinical clerkships in obstetrics and gynecology.

When I was a student at the University of Michigan during the 1940s, there were no problems in my rotation on the general medicine or surgical clerkships on male or female wards. The University Hospital's small obstetrics and gynecology service at the University Hospital in Ann Arbor, however, was inadequate to meet teaching needs of all the medical students. Students therefore customarily were divided into sections and rotated through that clerkship in a large hospital for women located in nearby Detroit. Since that hospital did not accept Blacks, the Black medical students were advised to make their own arrangements to do their clerkships anywhere in the nation in hospitals that would accept them. In 1945 I spent a month at Provident Hospital in Chicago, and while it was a productive month, I was the last Black student who had to endure this prejudicial arrangement. This practice continued until 1946, at which time the medical school arranged for Black students to remain in Ann Arbor for their clerkships. Until that change occurred, Blacks customarily spent a month usually at one of three hospitals, Harlem Hospital in New York City, Homer G. Phillips Hospital in St. Louis, or Provident Hospital in Chicago. These same hospitals at that time offered nearly half of all the internships considered to be both available and desirable for Blacks, the others being Montefiore Hospital in New York, Jersey City Medical Center, Cleveland City Hospital, and Wayne County General just outside Detroit, which first opened up in 1947 to another Black intern and me. These difficulties were encountered not only by Black men, but by Black women also. Nor were these exclusions limited to the medical student years. A Black woman obstetrician and gynecologist who was on the faculty of one of the Philadelphia medical schools told me that when she applied for residency training at one of the teaching hospitals in Philadelphia, just after World War II, she was notified by letter that she was not accepted, despite her qualifications, because her work as a resident on the obstetrics and gynecology service would require her to have intimate contact with patients. In that era, when color-caste was an accepted custom, Blacks as servants were allowed to have extremely close and intimate relations with Whites, including living with them in the same home, but intimacy as equals in social relations was not a normal expectation.

To what extent did these prejudices persist into later decades? A 1976 national study of women's preferences for the racial composition of medical facilities (Udry, Morris, and Bauman 1976) carried out in family planning clinics asked respondents whether they preferred to receive their medical care where the *(a)* patients, *(b)* nurses, or *(c)* doctors were (1) White and Black (2) all White, (3) all Black, or (4) did not matter.

In both 1969–70 and 1973–74, only 2 to 3.5 percent of Black women said they preferred medical facilities in which either patients, nurses, or doctors were all Black. Their attitudes were similar whether they were from the North or the South, and there were no differences by age or educational level. Black women either actively preferred racially integrated medical service programs (positive responses going from 30.0 percent in 1969 to 53.0 percent in 1973), or would passively accept them (responses that it didn't matter one way or the other changing from 68.0 percent in 1969 to 43.5 percent in 1973).

In both time periods, larger percentages of White women preferred to be treated in medical facilities where all patients were White. In the North this response was given by 11.0 percent in 1969, and 10.0 percent in 1973, in the South by 36.0 percent in 1969, and 19.0 percent in 1973. White women had slightly less preference for an all-White nursing staff (approximately 2.0 percentage points less than the preference for all-White patients). However, there was a high and persistent preference for all-White doctors: women from the North shifted from 37.0 percent to 27.0 percent by 1973, and in the South from 75.0 percent to 59.0 percent in 1973–74. A statement of active preference for racially integrated physician staff was obtained from White women from the North as follows: 16 percent in 1969, up to 27.0 percent by 1973. From the South: 6.0 percent in 1969 and increasing to 13.0 percent in 1973–74. While this suggests slight but definite improvement in receptivity to racially integrated medical facilities, it indicates how widespread the problem remained. Among White women who would passively accept integration, judging from their statement that the physician's race was not a matter of importance: the 1973 response in the North was 45.0 percent, in the South it was 28.0 percent. Thus, by 1973–74, three-fourths of White women from the North would to some degree accept a racially integrated medical staff, but this could be said of fewer than half of the southern White women. Furthermore, in 1973–74, White women from the South with some college education differed little from those who had less education.

Udry raised the possibility that more Black women might utilize medical services if they were racially integrated, but this might not be true for Whites. In commenting on this article, Cornely (1976) pointed out that, even though the improvement in racial attitudes seemed small, it was definitely favorable since it occurred in the short course of four years. Even more, he added, the negative social and public health costs of continued racial segregation are so considerable that a forthright public health policy position must be taken unequivocally in favor of promoting the continued racial integration of all medical staff and programs. In the 1950s, when Reitzes (1958) surveyed the pattern of racial desegregation in the medical field in selected major urban centers, he cited repeated instances in which the firmness of commitment on the part of White leadership was the necessary ingredient in opening up a hospital to Blacks as patients or professional staff members. Ordinarily, impoverished Blacks were most readily admitted to charity hospitals or wards; more difficult problems were encountered in the admission of Black patients who could pay to be admitted to a semiprivate room with a White patient. Similarly, Black nurses were more readily accepted on a hospital staff than Black physicians. The management of social and racial status has played and continues to play an unrecognized but important role in American medicine.

A question may be raised as to whether or not the rejection of Blacks as physicians in 1969–74 reflected prejudice, attitudinal and verbally expressed, or simply expressed the reality that White physicians were preferred because they had probably received better education and training. The crux of the affirmative action problem is that the discriminatory exclusion of Blacks can be justified endlessly by arguing that they are excluded not because they are Black, but because they are not as competently trained. In fact, only by removing the social institutional supports for racial inequality can we remove the phenomenon of institutionalized racism. These social hierarchical arrangements make it difficult for individuals to recognize their racial prejudice. As increasing number of Blacks are allowed to become physicians, and specialists, their social acceptance will occur, along with a perception of their equal competence as they become a part of a changed social reality. While it is true that such a future development will also possibly create a circumstance in which more Black patients will prefer all-Black medical facilities and an all-Black physician staff, opinion studies to date have shown that Blacks overwhelmingly favor a racially integrated society.

Blacks and Whites in the majority share a broad consensus on the value of a racially integrated and egalitarian society, but more Whites than Blacks believe that great progress has been made in recent decades, and Whites increasingly express a belief in these principles but "substantially less support for practices intended to implement principles of racial equality" (Jaynes and Williams 1989, chap. 3; Hochschild 1995, chap. 14 and appendix A). Increasing polarization and alienation particularly is being felt by the more affluent and well-educated Blacks, who feel more keenly a hardening of racial segregation and reduced opportunity within the past several decades, ironically since the 1954 Supreme Court decision, *Brown v. Board of Education* ended the "separate but equal" in principle but not in fact (Klinker and Smith 1999, chap. 9).

MINORITY ACCEPTANCE IN GME PROGRAMS

DEFINITION OF TERMS

In this review of affirmative action progress in graduate medical education, an attempt was made to demonstrate for the 1973–77 period the degree to which minority interns were accepted into GME programs in the northeastern, midwestern, western, and southern geographical regions of the nation. Hospitals included in this review are among the major teaching hospitals in the United States. The necessary criterion for including a hospital was that it had been selected by at least five interns from either the minority or the nonminority study sample in the 1973–77 time period. Almost all major and well-known postgraduate training programs associated with United States medical schools were included automatically by this procedure.

Some programs are listed as one, with the NIRMP and AMA data on graduate medical education programs recorded that way, even though they represent a cluster of several teaching hospitals. This is the case with the St. Louis University Group of Hospitals and the University of Utah affiliated hospitals, a group of nine hospitals listed as one training program.

The concept of minority acceptance rate expressed the degree to which a given hospital's training programs were chosen by individuals from our minority or nonminority study samples, each of which was comprised of approximately two thousand interns in the 1973–77 time period. Since roughly equal numbers of interns were included in each study sample, any given hospital would have been chosen in a 1:1 ratio if chance alone determined internship matches at that hospital. A hospital with an equal minority acceptance rate, therefore, would show roughly equal numbers of minority or nonminority interns (M:N ratios). Accordingly, examples of equal acceptance rates are M:N ratios of 5:5, 12:10, or 18:22, the numbers representing the actual numbers from the samples of minority (M) or nonminority (N) interns at that hospital. In those hospitals, minority and nonminority interns are defined as having had approximately equal chances of being selected.

High minority acceptance rates are defined as hospitals chosen by at least five minority interns, but with at least twice as many minority as nonminority interns. Thus, examples of high minority access rates (M > N) might be 5:2, 9:4, 30:10, again with actual numbers indicating the numbers of interns from each sample choosing that hospital. What this means is that minority interns had a definitely greater chance of being accepted than nonminority interns at that hospital. We cannot necessarily conclude, however, that such hospitals displayed the greatest affirmative action requirement activity. For example, if a given hospital's training positions were low in closeness of affiliation with a medical school, low in prestige rank, high in percentage of unfilled positions, and high in percentage of FMGs on the house staff, it would accept almost any minority or nonminority U.S. medical school graduate.

If the reverse of those conditions prevailed, the hospital would be high on the list of many applicants, and could therefore be highly selective. Hospitals with equal minority acceptance rates (M = N) are considered to be those in which minority and nonminority interns had equal chances of being accepted, depending on their statistical presence in the applicant pool. The presence of significant numbers of minority interns represented a decisive change from earlier decades during which minorities had been underrepresented at these hospitals. Since these hospitals are among those most sought after by both minority and nonminority interns, and they are more prestigious than others, an intentional affirmative action selection policy would have been necessary to produce this result.

Hospitals with low rates of minority acceptance may fall into that category either because little effort was made to attract minority interns, minority interns showed little interest or desire for such programs, or a combination of both. Absence or very low minority representation in an institution is often explained by a complete lack or dearth of qualified applicants. In the 1950s, when U.S. hospital desegregation began to occur, Reitzes observed that hospital leadership had to take the initiative and invite Blacks to apply, usually by informal conversation with qualified Black candidates, and these informal communications still play a major role. A Black physician joining the attending staff, or the house staff, following such an invitation would have a much more comfortable feeling than one who had gained his or her position only after court litigation. Understandably, under such adversarial circumstances a young Black physician could seldom function adequately, facing rejection from many White patients, as well as poor cooperation from nurses, colleagues, senior attending physicians, and administrators.

In 1945, the year I applied to hospitals for internship, I applied to the Wayne County General Hospital, the large county hospital just outside Detroit, which was a teaching hospital of Wayne State University Medical School. My application was prompted by conversations I had with Black medical students at Wayne and with Black physicians I knew socially. They had heard rumors that Wayne County was ready to accept a Black intern. On my graduation in 1946 I was accepted, along with another Black graduate from Meharry whose uncle held a high leadership position in Detroit politics. We were the first Blacks accepted and were warmly welcomed and assigned living quarters in the same building where other trainees lived.

It was through this same network of friends in Detroit that I learned of Dr. Viola Bernard's desire to help recruit Black physicians interested in pursuing training in psychiatry and psychoanalysis. A Black physician recently graduated from Wayne State and beginning his tour of duty in World War II was one of a group of doctors selected to take a six-month crash course to prepare them to become psychiatrists in the military service. The course was to be held at Camp Upton, and one of the instructors from Columbia University was Dr. Viola Bernard. In a discussion she had with my friend, the late Dr. Garnet Ice, he told her that his choice was to get residency training in surgery, which later he did. She told him to keep an eye open for a Black physician interested in her field and to have him or her come to New York to meet her for assistance. When I completed my first year of psychiatry training at Wayne County I realized I wanted to have further training. I wrote to Dr. Bernard, who invited me to come to New York, and on her advice I applied to the Long Island College of Medicine's hospitals for psychiatry residency training and to Columbia University for training in their psychoanalytic clinic for training and research.

REGIONAL REVIEWS

In the regions reviewed (Northeast, Midwest, West, and South), the states within a region are listed by rank from highest to lowest percentage of Black population. In order to follow a consistent format, that arrangement is followed even though in several western states the Hispanic population exceeds the Black. All state population statistics, given to the nearest tenth of a million, are from the 1970 census. Percentages of population for the various underrepresented minority groups are given to the nearest 0.05 percent. Those who are underrepresented both as medical students and as physicians are Blacks, Native Americans, and for Hispanics, of whom only Mexican Americans and mainland Puerto Ricans are included. These combined numbers of minority group persons within a state are another measure of political responsibility for the medically underserved within that jurisdiction. We recognize that federal government support to the states should compensate for the variations in internal resources available to meet the individual states needs. Obviously, a state with a very small minority group population would feel less compelled politically to develop a strong affirmative action medical program, although I show later that the degree of minority access to graduate medical education programs does not follow statewide or regional population-based needs alone.

Affirmative action can be inferred when the minority acceptance rate at a given training program is one minority acceptance to three nonminority acceptances or higher, such as 1:2 or 1:1 for example. In addition the graduate medical education programs must meet the additional requirement of being highly competitive and of high prestige because they meet at least three of the following four criteria: (1) they have a main (M) medical school affiliation, which means that both undergraduate medical students and postgraduate medical trainees are present; (2) they have a prestige rank of 1, 2, 3, or 4 (number 1 being best on a scale that went from 1 to 8, an informal ranking in use at Cornell during the 1970s); (3) they have fewer than 15 percent unfilled residency positions; and (4) they have fewer than 15 percent of their positions filled by foreign medical graduates (FMGs). Affirmative action GME programs so defined are indicated by an asterisk on tables 24, 25, 26, and 27, which follow. While this does not imply that all other hospitals did not exert strong affirmative action re-cruitment efforts, it is more difficult to identify such efforts from our data. Our only assumption is that for almost all of those hospitals, without as-terisks, becoming an accepted applicant would probably have been as great a problem either for minority or nonminority applicants.

NORTHEAST REGION

New York

Many major hospitals in New York have graduate medical education pro-grams that show a high rate of minority acceptance, as can be seen from table 24. They include large public general hospitals (like Harlem, Kings County, Bronx Municipal, and Bellevue) and some of the large voluntary hospitals (Roosevelt, St. Luke's, Mt. Sinai, and Brookdale). Most are lo-cated in neighborhoods with large minority populations, a few border on such neighborhoods, and the USPHS Hospital on Staten Island was at that time in an area of low minority group concentration. Since some of these hospitals (as shown by asterisk) were very much desired for intern-ships, and therefore highly competitive, it was immediately suggested that the stronger hospitals probably select only the stronger minority appli-cants, and that the weaker hospitals probably accept the weaker minority applicants. The weaker hospital programs are among those that most often must rely on FMG house staff. These hospitals also are important, how-ever, as service providers to minority and low-income groups.

Note that Harlem Hospital is not defined as an affirmative action GME recruiter despite the fact that no other hospital in the nation attracted so high a proportion of minority applicants. This is because Harlem does not meet the criteria for a highly competitive and high prestige hospital, which is attributed to the facts that over 15 percent of its residency positions usu-ally are unfilled and that more than 15 percent of those filled are occupied by foreign medical school graduates. This is true even though Harlem is one of the main teaching hospitals of Columbia University since both medical undergraduate students and postgraduate trainees are present and the programs are not only well run but are a major resource of medical care for central Harlem and its more than 90 percent Black and predom-inantly low-income community. It should be noted also that some of the minority residents choosing Harlem were among the top students in their class and note too that a small but significant number of nonminority residents also chose Harlem during the period of the 1970s.

Next, many hospitals in New York have equal minority acceptance rates. Here again, we can see strong evidence that minority candidates succeed in obtaining some of these most highly selective house staff positions, in hospitals associated with either private or public medical schools.

By our methodology, relatively few hospitals in New York could be categorized as falling into the group with low minority acceptance rates. Moreover, of the three hospitals in that category, none was classified with the most highly competitive group. The low minority presence in these hospitals probably was a reflection of low minority applicant interest rather than exclusion on the part of the hospitals. Perhaps it is relevant to note, however, that first-year undergraduate minority medical student enrollment at Albany Medical College also had been in the order of 1.0 percent for many years.

Generally, it can be seen that the pattern of affirmative action at the graduate medical education level closely parallels the record of undergraduate medical school admissions (the twenty-five preferred medical schools in the first column of table 14 are also the top twenty-five schools in production of graduates). It is noteworthy, however, that some medical centers were doing far more for affirmative action at the graduate medical education level than at the undergraduate medical student enrollment level. New York medical schools that provided affirmative action leadership at the GME level at the time of the study were Columbia Physicians and Surgeons, Albert Einstein, and New York University.

New Jersey

In the years under review, the Martland Medical Center was the major teaching hospital for the College of Medicine and Dentistry of New Jersey at Newark. While it is classified with the hospitals demonstrating equal minority acceptance rates (see table 24), the M:N ratio of 21:14 shows a tilt in favor of the minority group. Certainly this accords with the strong record of affirmative action at CMDNJ-Newark during the 1970s. Note that Martland Medical Center is not defined as an affirmative action GME recruiter for reasons identical to those for the Harlem Hospital Center. This takes nothing away from the fact that in other respects Martland has an exemplary overall affirmative action mission and accomplishment.

Following the Newark racial riots in 1967, many of the minority community demands were directed at the medical center. The old Martland plant at that time was to be replaced by a new university hospital building,

TABLE 24. Intern Selection Patterns in Northeastern Hospitals

State	Hospitals Showing High Minority Acceptance (M > N)		Hospitals Showing Equal Minority Acceptance (M = N)		Hospitals Showing Low Minority Acceptance (M < N)	
New York 11.9% Black 5.1% Hispanic 0.2% Native American	Harlem Columbia Physicians and Surgeons	95:6	*Montefiore Albert Einstein	22:14	Albany Medical Albany Medical College	2:15
	Kings County SUNY (Downstate)	27:10	NY Medical NY Medical	16:13	Long Island Jewish SUNY (Stonybrook)	1:6
	Brookdale NYU	14:7	*Presbyterian P&S Columbia P&S	11:6	Beth Israel Mt. Sinai	3:6
	Roosevelt Columbia Physicians and Surgeons	13:2	*New York Cornell	11:14		
	NYU NYU	10:0	St. Vincents NY Medical	7:7		
	*Bronx Municipal Albert Einstein	10:4	SUNY (Upstate) SUNY (Upstate)	7:10		
	*St. Lukes Columbia Physicians and Surgeons	10:5	Buffalo General SUNY (Buffalo)	5:3		
	*Mt. Sinai Mt. Sinai	9:3	Deaconess, Buffalo SUNY (Buffalo)	4:6		
	USPHS-Staten Island NY Medical	7:3	*Northshore Cornell	4:7		
	*Highland (Rochester) U. of Rochester	5:2	*Strong Memorial U. of Rochester	4:7		
	Bellevue NYU	5:1	U. of Rochester U. of Rochester	4:7		
New Jersey 10.7% Black 2.02% Hispanic			Martland Medical Center CMDNJ-Newark	21:14		
Pennsylvania 8.6% Black 0.46% Hispanic	Episcopal Temple	5:0	Thomas Jefferson Jefferson Medical	10:10	*U. of Pennsylvania Hospital U. of Pennsylvania	4:12
	Mercy Catholic Jefferson Medical	5:2	Temple Temple	9:7	*Hershey Pennsylvania State	2:6

State / Demographics	Hospital	Medical School	Ratio
	Presbyterian (U. of Pittsburgh)	Pittsburgh	9:12
	Children's	U. of Pennsylvania / Hahnemann / Jefferson	2:8
	Hahnemann	Hahnemann	5:8
	*Montefiore	Pittsburgh	5:6
Connecticut 6.0% Black 1.3% Hispanic	*Yale New Haven	Yale	18:18
	Hartford	U. of Connecticut	1:8
Massachusetts 3.1% Black 0.47% Hispanic	*Boston City	Boston University / Harvard	10:13
	*Beth Israel	Harvard	8:8
	*Mass. General	Harvard	6:9
	*Peter Bent Brigham	Harvard	5:8
	*New England Medical	Tufts	5:3
	*New England Deaconess	Harvard	4:5
New Hampshire 0.3% Black	Mary Hitchcock	Dartmouth	2:8
Vermont 0.2% Black	U. of Vermont Medical	U. of Vermont	0.6

Note: The name of the hospital is followed by the name of the medical school with which it is affiliated.

*An affirmative action hospital shows an acceptance ratio of at least 1:3 minority to nonminority ratio and meets the following criteria: (1) a main teaching hospital with both undergraduate medical students and postgraduate trainees, (2) a high prestige ranking according to the informal ranking system in use at Cornell during the 1970s, (3) fewer than 15% unfilled residency positions. (4) fewer than 15% foreign medical school house staff.

which opened in 1979, and new medical school buildings also were being planned. All of this new facility development necessitated relocation and rehousing of minority group tenants in the area. A very well organized and influential group of concerned citizens came into being and pressed for the following changes: increased minority admissions to the CMDNJ-Newark, increased admissions to its GME programs, increased minority faculty recruitment, increased hiring of minorities at higher levels of hospital staff, and the development of health services more directly relevant to the surrounding minority community's needs.

Much has been rumored about the excessive or inappropriate nature of community group pressure on academic admission or retention, as well as in hiring decisions. I have had discussions with several persons closely involved in the affairs of the school, and it would appear that despite obvious problems, a great number of positive achievements have been made at CMDNJ-Newark in response to community pressure. From 1970 to 1980, 15 percent or more minority students were admitted each year, and of those 96 percent graduated. Even though a large fraction of the students came from educationally disadvantaged backgrounds, support programs promoted their academic success. In the area of minority faculty recruitment, CMDNJ-Newark had three Blacks who were full professors, of whom two were clinical department heads. Many of the medical school graduates, both minority and nonminority, chose to remain in Newark to pursue their GME training at the medical center. Hospital hiring showed minority representation at all levels, and the executive director of the hospital was Black. Ambulatory health care programs, essentially a series of seven neighborhood based health centers, were operated directly by the Newark health department, while the medical center provided hospital backup support. Those ambulatory health care programs have been cited as one of the nation's most effective demonstrations that a high level of health care can be delivered to a neighborhood unable to attract solo practitioners. The effectiveness of these programs is shown, for example, in the improved prenatal and perinatal care that brought about a dramatic decline in infant mortality in the Newark Black population. Effective efforts to find care for patients early in the course of a disease were aimed at patients who suffer from chronic health problems, and the tuberculosis mortality rate was sharply reduced. By any fair judgment, CMDNJ-Newark was responding positively not only to the medical needs of Newark's Black community, which is 54 percent of the population, but to the city of Newark and that part of their state as a whole ("Health Care in Newark" 1978, 1979; Miller et al. 1981).

Pennsylvania

Another more troublesome scenario was enacted in several major urban centers, one of the most notable of which was Philadelphia. Philadelphia General Hospital, once the oldest and best of its kind, was closed in 1976. Since many persons used the hospital inappropriately as a substitute for ambulatory health care services, the hospital was to be replaced by several ambulatory health care clinics located in minority and low-income neighborhoods.

Minority groups are aware that if they lose their neighborhood hospital, they risk losing immediate or definite access to hospital care, and they have no assurance of receiving any of the promised substitute service programs. Because no funds were appropriated to develop a tracking system ("Closing of Philadelphia General Hospital" 1978; JRB Associates 1979), it was not possible to document how many persons who had been served by Philadelphia General Hospital no longer received necessary hospital care once it closed. Particularly vulnerable were patients without financial resources or coverage, patients with problems of substance abuse, or patients involuntarily admitted for psychiatric problems. Our study shows, however, that in the whole 1973–77 period of review, when the hospital's GME programs were being closed, only one minority intern went into that hospital. Losing that once great hospital as a magnet was apparently not compensated for by the other GME training programs operated by the five Philadelphia medical schools. Undergraduate medical education opportunity was, therefore, a considerably greater success than was affirmative action at the GME level. While the medical schools in Pennsylvania produced 152 minority graduates, that state attracted only ninety-seven minority interns in the same 1973–77 time period (see table 15). Table 24 shows that the only hospitals in Pennsylvania that had high minority acceptance rates were the relatively weak Episcopal and Mercy hospitals, both of which are located in the inner city.

Connecticut, Massachusetts, New Hampshire, Vermont

Two of these states exemplify the role of university teaching hospital's leadership in affirmative action at the GME level; the records of Harvard and Yale are shown in table 24. Harvard very early assumed a leadership role in the sustained admission of minority students to its medical school, having admitted more than 12 percent each year throughout the 1970s. We note that minority candidates apparently had equal chances of being selected for GME training at Harvard's affiliated hospitals, although these are among the most competitive placements. It is also known that Harvard's minority faculty recruitment was and continues to be ahead of most other schools. The absence of major hospitals showing high minority acceptance rates in any of these states probably reflects the lack of large concentrations of minority group populations. Harvard and Yale traditionally, however, draw students from the nation as a whole and are less bound by statewide perspectives.

It should be noted that the Harvard achievement was not made without turmoil. A faculty member's editorial in the *New England Journal of Medicine* in 1976 (Davis 1976) bemoaned the lowering of standards brought about by the admission of unqualified minority students. The Harvard faculty and administration asserted overwhelmingly that their minority students were qualified, including the student whose graduation had prompted the faculty member's editorial dissent. (Both pro and con assertions as stated in this editorial were unaccompanied by data.)

The low minority acceptance rates to GME programs under the direction of the University of Connecticut, Dartmouth, and the University of Vermont are best understood as a result of the very small Black populations in their surrounding areas, or in their undergraduate medical schools.

THE MIDWEST

Illinois and Michigan

Illinois and Michigan demonstrated similar profiles of minority acceptance in GME training programs: the hospitals were divided between those that showed high or low rates of minority acceptance, with relatively few hospitals in the equal acceptance range. Most of the major university teaching hospitals appear to be open to minorities, although several do not appear to be equally available (table 25).

Historically, Illinois, particularly Chicago, played an important role in the desegregation of medicine in the nation, and has followed an interesting course of evolutionary change. As Reitzes outlined these events (1958, on Chicago, 103–33; Detroit, 149–68; St. Louis, 256–69; Los Angeles, 180–89; Atlanta, 272–94; New Orleans, 295–315), the first major achievement came in 1929, through the leadership of Dr. Franklin C. McLean, head of medicine and of medical clinics at the University of Chicago and dean for many years. He obtained financial support, principally from the Rosenwald Fund, to strengthen a Black hospital, Provident Hospital, on Chicago's South Side, not only to meet the needs of Black patients but also to provide clinical training for Black undergraduate medical students and postgraduates seeking training in the medical specialties. With Dr. McLean's resignation from the Provident board in 1932, that hospital's affiliation with the University of Chicago gradually weakened and by 1944 was ended.

Provident continued to serve Black patients exclusively but also came to have an almost completely Black physician staff, and although that had not been its original intent, the very existence of Provident reduced the professional interchange between Black and White physicians and slowed Chicago's progress in the racial integration of medicine.

By the mid-1950s 26.2 percent of the 226 Black physicians in Chicago were board certified, but only 7.1 percent had affiliations with predominantly White hospitals. Black physicians who had had postgraduate training in predominantly White hospitals were most likely to obtain attending privileges at such hospitals. Thus, 8 of the 38 Blacks trained at White hospitals (21.1 percent) had such appointments, while of 50 Blacks trained at a Black hospital, such as Provident, only 3 percent had attending privileges at White hospitals.

Cook County Hospital, which originally was established to care for the medically indigent, was the chief hospital care resource for Chicago's Blacks. In 1955, 60 percent of all Black babies born in hospitals were delivered at Cook County. Black physicians found themselves in a difficult, competitive situation, since Provident was almost the only hospital available for them to admit their middle-income Black patients. Prosperous and well-educated Black patients, like others similarly situated, preferred to be admitted to high-prestige hospitals and therefore usually sought out White physicians and hospitals if possible. So segregated was hospital care in Chicago in the mid-1950s that many Black workers, whose union health coverage plans paid for hospital care, found it impossible to gain admission to a voluntary hospital. Special arrangements, therefore, were made by means of which Cook County not only would accept indigent Black patients, but Blacks who could pay or who had third-party coverage as well. Quite clearly by the late 1950s in Chicago, Provident, as an all-Black hospital with no major university connection, had outlived its initial purpose and mission. Provident has played no role in GME for Blacks since the late 1950s. Only an opening up of the other major hospitals offered any hope for improved opportunities either for Black patients or for Black physicians in the Chicago area.

The fact that Detroit, even though it contained several privately owned and operated all-Black hospitals, never had Black hospitals involved in undergraduate or postgraduate medical education, probably stimulated more consistent integrationist movement in that area. As Reitzes (1958) illustrated, in the mid-1950s, of forty-seven hospitals in the Detroit metropolitan area, seventeen did not normally admit Blacks; the remaining thirty admitted them often in significant numbers, although twenty of those reported some degree of racial segregation in bed assignment. Physicians fared better than

TABLE 25. Intern Selection Patterns in Midwestern Hospitals

State	Hospitals Showing High Minority Acceptance (M > N)	Hospitals Showing Equal Minority Acceptance (M = N)	Hospitals Showing Low Minority Acceptance (M < N)
Illinois 12.8% Black 2.2% Hispanic	Cook County — 48:12 U. of Chicago U. of Illinois Northwestern U. *U. of Chicago — 24:9 U. of Chicago Michael Reese — 20:4 U. of Chicago U. of Illinois Northwestern U. Rush Presbyterian — 13:6 Rush Medical College Mercy Hospital Medical — 6:1 U. of Illinois Northwestern U.	U. of Illinois Affiliate — 17:10 U. of Illinois	Loyola U. Affiliate — 1:6 Loyola U. — 1:5 Childrens Memorial Northwestern
Michigan 11.2% Black 0.8% Hispanic	Wayne State U. Affiliate — 31:11 Wayne State U. Henry Ford — 24:5 U. of Michigan Hurley, Flint — 18:2 U. of Michigan Michigan State Childrens — 6:0 Wayne State Grace — 5:1 Wayne State *Southwest Michigan (AHEC) — 5:1 U. of Michigan St. John — 5:2 Wayne State	Providence (Southfield) — 9:6 U. of Michigan Wayne State	*U. of Michigan Affiliate — 9:27 U. of Michigan William Beaumont — 1:7 Wayne State Butterworth — 1:5 (Grand Rapids) U. of Michigan Michigan State St. Joseph Mercy — 2:7 Wayne State U. of Michigan
Missouri 10.3% Black	Homer G. Phillips — 5:0 Washington U.	*Barnes, St. Louis — 7:9 Washington U. St. Louis U. — 7:11 St. Louis U.	U. of Missouri — 1:13 U. of Missouri (Columbia)

State / Demographics	Hospital — Medical School	Ratio	Hospital — Medical School	Ratio	Hospital — Medical School	Ratio
			St. Louis Childrens — Washington U.	6:9		
			Kansas City General — U. of Missouri (Kansas City)	5:7		
			*Jewish, St. Louis — Washington U.	5:5		
Ohio 9.1% Black 0.4% Hispanic	*Veterans Administration — Case Western	11:1	*Cincinnati General — U. of Cincinnati	18:14	Mt. Carmel — Ohio State	2:7
	Cleveland Clinics — Case Western	7:3	Case Western Reserve — Case Western	15:9	Akron General Affiliate — Ohio State	0:7
	Mt. Sinai — Case Western	5:0	Cleveland Metropolitan General — Case Western	10:6	*Riverside Methodist — Ohio State	0:5
	Case Western		Ohio State U. — Ohio State	4:7		
			Akron City — Ohio State	4:7		
Indiana 6.9% Black 0.8% Hispanic			*Indiana U. Medical — Indiana U.	21:19		
			Methodist — Indiana U.	10:12		
Kansas 4.8% Black 1.0% Hispanic					*U. Kansas Medical Center — U. of Kansas	3:6
					St. Francis — U. of Kansas	1:5
Wisconsin 2.9% Black					Medical College Wisconsin Affiliate — Medical College Wisconsin	5:11
					U. of Wisconsin Affiliate — U. of Wisconsin	2:13
Nebraska 2.7% Black					Creighton University Affiliate — Creighton U.	4:9
					*U. of Nebraska Affiliate — U. of Nebraska	0:9
Iowa 1.2% Black					*U. of Iowa Hospital — U. of Iowa	3:12
Minnesota 0.9% Black 0.6% Indian					*Mayo — Mayo Medical	8:18
					*Hennipen County — U. of Minnesota	0:7

Note: The name of the hospital is followed by the name of the medical school with which it is affiliated.

*An affirmative action hospital of highest degree, meeting the following criteria: (1) a main teaching hospital with both undergraduate medical students and postgraduate trainees, (2) a high prestige ranking according to the informal ranking system in use at Cornell during the 1970s, (3) fewer than 15% unfilled residency positions, (4) fewer than 15% foreign medical school house staff.

in Chicago; of Detroit's 160 Black physicians, 15.6 percent had attending privileges at predominantly White hospitals. Of the 24 who had done residency training at White Hospitals, 54.4 percent had such appointments; and of the 64 whose residency training had been done at Black hospitals, 18.7 percent had attending privileges at predominantly White hospitals.

With that perspective, our findings for the 1973–77 period show that in Illinois, and especially Chicago, considerable improvements are apparent. The big question remains whether the demise of Cook County Hospital would seriously diminish GME opportunities for Blacks and other underrepresented minorities. It is a positive sign that the major academic medical centers in Chicago are demonstrating a high and promising degree of acceptance of minority candidates.

In the Detroit area, the leadership role of Wayne State University's affiliated hospitals suggested that in the future a group of highly trained Black physicians would be available.

Missouri

Like Provident Hospital in Chicago, Homer G. Phillips Hospital in St. Louis offered one of the best internships available for Blacks in the 1930s and 1940s. The hospital was named for a Black civil rights lawyer, who in the 1930s led the fight to have the city build a hospital to which Blacks would be admitted. As Reitzes (1958) noted, this hospital succeeded in maintaining a strong university affiliation and a strong racially integrated physician staff far longer than Provident. In his position as chief of staff for Phillips, Dr. Robert Elman, who was also chairman of the Department of Surgery at Washington University School of Medicine, assumed primary responsibility for the quality of the GME training program at Phillips. Although he was White, his leadership was accepted by physicians of both races, and appointments of heads of clinical services were made on a basis of merit. It has been estimated that of all Black physicians practicing in the United States in the 1950s, 20 percent completed their GME-1 year at Homer G. Phillips, and half of all Black ophthalmologists were trained at Phillips. Almost all the Black physicians in St. Louis had chosen to remain after completing their training there ("Homer G. Phillips Hospital" 1976).

In the early 1960s, as GME opportunities for Blacks began to open up elsewhere, the importance of Homer G. Phillips as a training center declined. Even though the Department of Surgery at Washington University continued to maintain a vital interest in the Phillips surgery training program's strength, the medical school departmental connections generally weakened. In the 1973–77 period of our study the affiliation with Washington University was limited in type, but by 1977 Phillips did not offer places in the NIRMP match. For several years it had great difficulty at-tracting applicants. In fact, by 1979, Phillips was no longer operated as an acute care hospital, but only as an outpatient clinic and emergency room as a branch of the other major public general hospital in St. Louis.

In 1976, the hospital leadership at Phillips, arguing for the hospital's survival, pointed out that in fifteen years not more than five Black physi-cians had opened practices in St. Louis. Our findings in the 1973–77 pe-riod show no really major hospital training programs to which minority candidates had high rates of acceptance, and only modest numbers were enrolled in academic medical center programs to which minorities have equal acceptance. Only a fraction of minority residents who completed training from those academic centers remained in the St. Louis area. A Black physician who practices in the St. Louis area told me that only two Black residents completing training at local university centers in the pre-ceding few years had decided to stay in that city to practice. He thought that despite strong Black political opinion in favor of reviving Homer G. Phillips, there was little likelihood that its former strength could be re-vived, or that a climate of opinion could permit the dominant role once played by Washington University even if it were willing to do so. Note that the prestigious Barnes and Jewish Medical Centers both associated with Washington University are affirmative action GME recruiters.

Ohio and Indiana

Of states in the Midwest, Ohio showed a promising profile for the pres-ence of minority candidates in GME training programs, and a very con-siderable role of leadership was provided by Case Western Reserve Med-ical School. Indiana, through Indiana University, showed a picture of definite affirmative action recruitment.

Kansas, Wisconsin, Nebraska, Iowa, Minnesota

Kansas contains a substantial Black population. Nonetheless, it had a low level of minority acceptance to its major GME training programs. The other midwestern states listed had a low presence of minority residents, and this is also a pattern shown in undergraduate medical student enroll-ment, both of which are largely explained demographically.

THE WEST

Texas

Sometimes considered more southern than western, Texas was placed with the West primarily because of its population characteristics (table 26).

TABLE 26. Intern Selection Patterns in Western Hospitals

State	Hospitals Showing High Minority Acceptance (M > N)		Hospitals Showing Equal Minority Acceptance (M = N)		Hospitals Showing Low Minority Acceptance (M < N)	
Texas 12.5% Black 14.5% Hispanic 0.2% Native American	U. Texas Affiliate System (Houston) U. of Texas (Houston)	12:6	*Baylor U. Affiliate Baylor U.	40:27	U. of Texas Medical Branch (Galveston) U. of Texas (Galveston)	5:21
			*U. of Texas (San Antonio) (San Antonio)	19:20		
	Memorial Medical Center (Corpus Christi) No academic affiliation	7:0	U. of Texas (San Antonio) U. of Texas (Dallas) U. of Texas (Southwestern)	13:12	Baylor U. Medical Baylor U. Methodist (Dallas) U. of Texas (Southwestern)	0:17
			J. P. Smith U. of Texas (Southwestern)	8:6		
California 7.0% Black 9.3% Hispanic 0.5% Native American	*LA County USC U. of Southern California	74:38	*UC (San Francisco) UC San Francisco	17:11	UC Davis UC Davis	2:15
	Martin Luther King U. of California	71:3	*UC San Diego UC San Diego	14:12	St. Marys UC San Francisco	1:8
	*LA County Harbor General UCLA U. of California (Irvine)	32:10	Highland General UC San Diego	12:8		
	Children's North California UC San Francisco Stanford	7:1	Valley Medical Center (Fresno) UC San Francisco	12:7		
	*Loma Linda U. Loma Linda U.	7:1	*Stanford Stanford	10:7		
	*Kaiser LA U. of Southern California	6:1	*San Francisco General UC San Francisco	9:9		
	*Children's LA U. of Southern California UC Irvine	6:1	VA Center (Wordsworth) UCLA	6:6		
	Loma Linda		San Joaquin General UC Davis UC San Francisco	5:5		
	Santa Barbara General Kern General UCLA	5:1	*Cedars Sinai UCLA	5:5		
		5:1				

State	Demographics	Hospital / Medical School	Ratio
Oklahoma	6.7% Black 0.6% Hispanic 3.8% Native American	U. of Oklahoma Health U. of Oklahoma	7:10
Washington	2.1% Black 1.0% Hispanic 1.0% Native American	*U. of Washington Affiliate U. of Washington	8:16
Colorado	3.0% Black 4.8% Hispanic 0.4% Native American	*U. of Colorado Affiliate U. of Colorado	19:24
		St. Joseph	0:5
Arizona	3.0% Black 13.6% Hispanic 5.4% Native American	*U. of Arizona Affiliate U. of Arizona	8:8
		Maricopa County U. of Arizona	5:6
		UC San Francisco	5:3
		Good Samaritan U. of Arizona	5:3
		St. Joseph Medical U. of Arizona	5:3
		Tucson Medical U. of Arizona	2:6
Oregon	1.3% Black 0.6% Hispanic 0.6% Native American	U. of Oregon Health U. of Oregon	1:9
New Mexico	1.9% Black 11.8% Hispanic 7.2% Native American	U. of New Mexico Affiliate U. of New Mexico	5:3
Utah	0.6% Black 1.4% Hispanic 1.1% Native American	*U. of Utah Affiliate	6:13

Note: The name of the hospital is followed by the name of the medical school with which it is affiliated.

*An affirmative action hostgraduate hospital of highest degree, meeting the following criteria: (1) a main teaching hospital with both undergraduate medical students and postgraduate trainees, (2) a high prestige ranking according to the informal ranking system in use at Cornell during the 1970s, (3) fewer than 15% unfilled residency positions, (4) fewer than 15% foreign medical school house staff.

Texas shows a favorable balance in its general profile of minority acceptance to GME training programs. Among all states, it ranked fifth in production of minority medical school graduates and also in numbers of minority interns attracted to GME programs within that state (see chap. 4, table 15). Texas ranked eighth among the states in numbers of Black interns; second (behind California) in Mexican American interns; and ninth in numbers of Puerto Ricans.

In the current review of minority acceptance in major academic center GME programs, both of the University of Texas campuses and Baylor University were successfully attracting and training minority candidates.

California

California's profile of minority acceptance to GME programs was almost identical to that of New York state. However, if we look only at the number of highly competitive GME programs to which minority candidates had higher acceptance rates, California and New York both had five such programs, but California's programs included 125 minority interns compared to New York's 39. Similarly, both states had five GME programs in the equal acceptance category: California had 55 minority interns and New York had 52. The major academic medical centers, both public and private, were well represented in both high rates and equal rates of minority acceptance in both New York and California. Few GME programs in either state appeared to be relatively closed to minorities.

In 1958, Reitzes found 121 Black physicians in Los Angeles, but their rate of increase in the prior decade showed a larger percentage increase than in any American city. In that same year, Blacks had no particular problems in being admitted to hospitals as patients: only four of forty hospitals polled by the Los Angeles County Medical Association stated they did not accept Blacks. Black physicians were also found to be able to obtain hospital appointments more directly in line with the extent of their training, and Blacks trained in Black hospitals did not encounter greater difficulty in becoming attending physicians than Blacks trained in predominantly White hospitals. Since training opportunities only opened up after World War II, few Black physicians were trained as specialists. Again, Reitzes believed that the absence of a Black hospital in Los Angeles promoted racial integration.

In our review of the 1973–77 time period, it would appear that the development of postgraduate training programs at the Martin Luther King Medical Center in the Watts section of Los Angeles, which attracts minority candidates almost exclusively, had not retarded the acceptance of many other minority candidates applying to the predominantly White university teaching hospitals. This was a parallel development to that seen in New

York, where Harlem Hospital attracts large proportions of minority trainees, although other minority trainees seek out other programs. It is the presence of a strong link to a major university that makes these programs viable and popular both at Martin Luther King and at Harlem. What also is noteworthy is that minority candidates in California and New York were not limited to an essentially segregated training setting.

Oklahoma, Colorado, Arizona, New Mexico

These states provided minority candidates equal acceptance to the major university-linked GME programs.

Oregon and Utah

Low concentrations of minority people probably accounted for their low representation in these GME programs.

THE SOUTH

District of Columbia

Howard University's main GME training programs at Freedman's Hospital are not in the NIRMP match, because of traditional attitudes developed during earlier decades when their graduates were excluded from most GME programs. For that reason, table 27 understates the GME training available to minority candidates in the District of Columbia. By any measure there will be a secure future supply of well-trained Black physicians in this area.

Mississippi, Georgia, Maryland, Delaware

These states demonstrated that even in the South, some of the major university teaching hospital GME programs provided equal opportunity in acceptance of minority candidates. Many of the most competitive high-prestige programs in these states were open to minorities. Table 27 indicates that both the Georgetown and the George Washington University Hospitals are affirmative action GME recruiters.

Reitzes reported that in 1958, there were only thirty-six Black physicians in Atlanta, down from forty-two in 1938, even though the Black population was steadily increasing in those years. None of the Black physicians in 1958 was board certified. Grady Hospital at that time was segregated, with separate Black and White divisions, and Blacks were not accepted in the GME training programs. Not surprisingly, 70 percent of Atlanta Blacks used White physicians, and wealthy Blacks tended either to use White physicians or to travel to New York, Chicago, or St. Louis for treatment by Black physicians. Emory University's GME programs were open

TABLE 27. Intern Selection Patterns in Southern Hospitals

State	Hospitals Showing High Minority Acceptance (M > N)	Hospitals Showing Equal Minority Acceptance (M = N)	Hospitals Showing Low Minority Acceptance (M < N)
District of Columbia 71.1% Black 0.2% Hispanic	DC General 26:2 Howard Georgetown 12:3 Childrens George Washington Howard 10:2 Washington Hospital Center George Washington 5:0 St. Elizabeth George Washington	*Georgetown U. 11:6 Georgetown U. *George Washington U. 7:7 George Washington	
Mississippi 36.8% Black 0.2% Indian		*U. of Mississippi Hospitals 12:17	
South Carolina 30.5% Black			Richland Memorial 3:7 Medical U. of South Carolina
Louisiana 29.8% Black 0.3% Hispanic	USPHS 7:0 Tulane	Charity Hospital Louisiana 29:18 Louisiana State U.	Confederate Memorial 1:7 Louisiana State U. (Shreveport) Ochsner 1:6 Louisiana State U. Tulane E. K. Long 1:5 Louisiana State U. (Baton Rouge)
Alabama 26.2% Black			*U. Alabama Medical Center 3:10
Georgia 25.9% Black 0.2% Hispanic	Emory U. Affiliate 5:1 Emory U.	*Grady Memorial 37:23 Emory U. *Eugene Talmadge 13:12 Medical College Georgia	

State / Demographics	Hospital (Medical school)	Ratio(s)
North Carolina — 22.2% Black, 0.2% Hispanic, 0.9% Native American	*Duke U. Medical (Duke)	12:29
	*NC Memorial (U. North Carolina)	8:21
	NC Baptist (Bowman Gray)	1:18
	*Charlotte Memorial (U. North Carolina)	1:14
Virginia — 18.5% Black, 0.2% Hispanic	*Medical College of Virginia (Medical College of Virginia)	14:16
	U. of Virginia Affiliate (U. of Virginia)	1:6
	Roanoke Memorial (U. of Virginia)	0:7
Arkansas — 18.3% Black	U. of Arkansas Medical (U. of Arkansas)	6:14
Tennessee — 15.8% Black	Vanderbilt U. Affiliate (Vanderbilt)	2:20
	Baptist Memorial (U. of Tennessee)	1:8
Florida — 15.3% Black, 0.7% Hispanic	University Hospital Jacksonville (U. of Florida)	8:3 / 12:13
	Wm. Shands (U. of Florida)	6:12
	U. of Southern Florida Affiliate (U. of Southern Florida)	1:8
	Pensacola Ed. Pr. (U. of Florida)	1:5
Maryland — 14.3% Black, 0.3% Hispanic	USPHS (Baltimore) (U. of Maryland)	6:0 / 17:9
	Baltimore City (U. of Maryland)	6:1 / 16:15
	*Johns Hopkins (Johns Hopkins)	
Delaware — 14.3% Black, 0.6% Hispanic	Wilmington Medical Center (Jefferson Medical College)	8:2
Kentucky — 7.2% Black	U. of Louisville (U. of Louisville)	6:9
	U. of Kentucky Medical (U. of Kentucky)	0:16

Note: The name of the hospital is followed by the name of the medical school with which it is affiliated.

*An affirmative action hospital of highest degree, meeting the following criteria: (1) a main teaching hospital with both undergraduate medical students and postgraduate trainees, (2) a high prestige ranking according to the informal ranking system in use at Cornell during the 1970s, (3) fewer than 5% unfilled residency positions, (4) fewer than 15% foreign medical school house staff.

to minority candidates, whose acceptance rates were above average. The state of Georgia as a whole attracted many minority interns, sixty-one from our sample, but the state's medical schools produced only twenty-one minority medical school graduates (see chap. 4, table 15). Affirmative action succeeded more dramatically at the GME level, but it is this level that will insure a future supply of Black physicians in the Atlanta area.

Louisiana, Florida, Virginia and Kentucky showed less favorable patterns of minority acceptance, with a particular tendency for the most desirable programs to be relatively closed to minorities.

New Orleans had only thirty Black physicians in 1958, although there had been thirty-seven in 1938, even though the Black population had grown by almost 40 percent in the same period (Reitzes 1958). Only one of these Black physicians was board certified. Even though we found in the 1973–77 period that many of Louisiana's prime GME training programs still were closed to Blacks, some of their better programs were open. Louisiana medical schools graduated twenty-nine minority students from our 1973–77 sample, but attracted thirty-six interns in all, again showing greater progress at the GME level.

South Carolina, Alabama, North Carolina, Arkansas, Tennessee

The presence of Meharry Medical College in Nashville, whose GME programs were not included in the NIRMP, leads to an understatement of GME training opportunity for Blacks in the Nashville/Tennessee area. This probably cannot account for the low minority acceptance to GME training programs at Vanderbilt.

States such as South Carolina, Alabama, and Arkansas were perhaps not surprising in their small recruitment success, which is in line with their undergraduate medical student enrollment effort.

North Carolina's poor showing in GME programs was decidedly less favorable than its record of undergraduate medical student enrollment. Medical schools in North Carolina graduated forty-three minorities from our study sample in the 1973–77 period, but the state attracted only twenty-six interns (see chap. 4, table 15). Looking, as in table 15, only at the GME-1 enrollment in the major academic medical centers in North Carolina, we see that minority applicants fared less well than in any other state with several strong medical schools.

We observed a reduced level of minority acceptance to the stronger GME training programs for the whole southern region. The pattern, however, is variable and by no means monolithic. Particular mention should be made of Georgia, a state solely in the tradition of the Deep South, yet one in which both private and public medical schools have opened up their programs. Both Duke University in North Carolina and Johns Hopkins in Maryland indicate that the great private university teaching hospitals in the South are affirmative action GME recruiters.

A LOOK AT PROGRESS OVERALL

Progress was being made in acceptance of minority physicians, especially Blacks, to GME training programs from which they were previously excluded. Reitzes raised the possibility in the 1950s that the existence of a strong Black hospital in a given city could retard the further development of racially integrated medical facilities and programs. This would be likely to occur, he believed, under the following set of circumstances: (1) there was little commitment on the part of White or Black medical leadership to the benefits of racial integration, (2) there was no commitment to the importance of maintaining a racially integrated staff of physicians, even if all patients served were Black, and (3) there was no strong and sustained affiliation with a major university medical center. I basically agree with the soundness of those views and believe they are still relevant today.

However, important developments since the beginning of desegregation in the 1950s, demonstrate how difficult it will be to achieve integration in the decades to come. Public opinion among White Americans remains either opposed to, ambivalent toward, or not forthrightly committed to racial integration in our national life or to the social benefits that racial equality would contribute to the country as a whole. The findings reported by Udry and his colleagues, on White attitudes toward the use of racially integrated medical facilities and services, parallel studies that reveal the reluctance of Whites to live in racially integrated neighborhoods or in other such intimate social relationships (Rothbart 1976)—a state of affairs that has persisted. Neighborhoods in many urban areas are still undergoing changes from almost all White to almost all Black, a state of affairs that will continue in the absence of dramatic changes in federal urban public policy. As neighborhoods become all Black, they lose their ability to maintain a strong middle class and gradually are abandoned by strong schools, businesses, hospitals, and other necessary social institutions.

Likewise, strong Black institutions such as hospitals, businesses, and churches, face survival problems similar to those faced by strong White hospitals or other institutions located in all-Black neighborhoods. Federal, state, and local planning and financing will be required to maintain an acceptable level of health, education, social, and other services within these Black neighborhoods that are created by White flight. What is needed is a strong public commitment to be rid of the problems brought on by the racial segregation of neighborhoods; we hear too many suggestions that we should get rid of Blacks, rather than the problems that are thrust upon them. Given the current climate of national public opinion, it would be unwise to advocate the elimination of hospitals located in Black neighborhoods, in anticipation that Blacks would thereby automatically be accepted equally, either as patients or as professionals, in the predominantly White hospitals located in predominantly White neighborhoods.

By a fortunate happenstance, many of our high-prestige universities, medical schools, and medical centers now find themselves located within or near almost totally Black inner-city neighborhoods. The fact that it would be insupportably expensive to relocate these institutions creates a strong pressure for them to remain where they are, and to assume a role of leadership in the redevelopment of their surrounding communities. This could not occur, however, with a paternalistic model of White leadership, which was appropriate in earlier decades when Reitzes gave it praise. Today, a pattern of genuine collaboration and shared leadership with the minority community is the more acceptable model. Responsibility for taking initiative in this collaboration would have to be taken by Whites who still hold the balance of power in their hands.

A similar quandary concerns the wisdom of maintaining a public general hospital system originally designed for the medically indigent alongside a private voluntary hospital system for paying patients. At first glance, it would appear in the social interest to have only one hospital system for all people. Such a desirable end does not, however, necessarily require elimination of the public general hospitals of our large cities. Patients served by these hospitals have often found them to be their only port of entry to the health care system. Further, because they have been so vital a component in the education and training of undergraduate and graduate medical students, patients have usually received high-quality care. Traditionally, in other words, the public general hospitals have been a major resource for removing social class barriers to hospital care. The Commission on Public General Hospitals (1978) and other experts have concluded that public hospitals should, however, be divested of their image of being hospitals only for the poor (Ginzberg et al. 1979). All social classes should be served and new services developed and diversified to provide hospital care that the private voluntary hospitals would find financially unprofitable. Such services for all would include, among others, emergency and trauma care, health education and preventive programs, neighborhood-based primary and ambulatory care, long-term care, and the handling of difficult medical-social problems such as substance abuse and certain psychiatric disorders.

PART III

VII. Thirty-Year Progress Report

GEOGRAPHIC LOCATION OF PRACTICE AND MEDICAL SPECIALTY DISTRIBUTION

METHODOLOGY

MEASURES

THIS CHAPTER PRESENTS thirty-year follow-up data on the medical careers of approximately 90 percent of the minority and nonminority medical students in the baseline data study group. Students were admitted to medical schools in the four-year period beginning in 1969 and graduated in the years 1973 through 1977.

The baseline data for the 4,134 subjects in the initial study were coded by an expert in market research. A code book was developed by a researcher on my staff at the Harlem Hospital Center Psychiatry Department, who also reviewed and corrected the data set. The following data were coded: unique identifying number, year of graduation from medical school, ethnicity, sex, National Medical Fellowship status (whether they applied for, and, if so, were awarded, an NMF grant); medical school code, and postgraduate training code.

Follow-up data on medical career were obtained from the 1994 edition of the *American Medical Directory* (AMA 1994) and coded as defined in the code book: vital status, zip code of primary office address, medical school of graduation, year of medical license, primary and secondary self-designated specialty, type of practice, and first and second American specialty board certification.

Machine-readable data from the 1990 full U.S. zip code areas from the Census of Population and Housing were obtained. (Wendy Treadwell, coordinator, Center for Machine Readable Data, University of Minnesota, provided data from the 1990 full U.S. zip code areas from the Census of Population and Housing, 1990. Summary Tape File 3B was linked with the zip codes of the 3,788 respondents with zip code data.) These data were

linked with zip codes for the 3,788 physicians who supplied that information for the medical directory. No substantial bias was created by missing
census data.

Using data from the *Statistical Abstract of the USA 1991,* our researcher
ascertained that there were twenty-three cities with populations of 500,000
or more as measured by the 1990 census. Using the *Rand McNally Zip Code
Finder, 1995,* the zip codes for those twenty-three cities were given study
codes. We defined each of those as a "big city" in describing the location of
the medical practice. Demographic data for total populations residing in
zip codes are derived from the 1990 census.

Census data included not only the total population residing in the zip
code area but also persons who are African American or Hispanic and
whose average household income is less than $5,000; $5,000 to $10,000;
$10,000 to $15,000; more than $15,000. This allowed us to characterize
practice locations at varying proportions of ethnicity and income levels.

Of the 4,134 subjects in the baseline data set, 316 (7.6 percent) were lost
to follow-up, and 365 (8.8 percent) had addresses in zip codes with no population (e.g. post office boxes, possibly districts zoned as nonresidential,
etc.). Review of the distributions of these missing data led us to conclude
that no significant bias was introduced by this finding. Thus we omitted
from analyses those physicians with zip codes but no census data where
population characteristics were relevant.

STATISTICAL METHODS

The study data set was analyzed using standard statistical methods (e.g.
cross-tabulation of categorical variables using chi-square and adjusted cell
residuals to assess whether observed distributions were significantly different than expected by chance alone; *t*-tests; and analysis of variance).

SCALES

The following ethnic groups were defined: African American (AA); other
minority (OM); Native American (AI); and Hispanic (HI), subdivided
into Mexican (MEX) and Puerto Rican from the U.S. mainland (PR).
Also defined was the general category of all nonminority (NM) and all minority (M) physicians.

Within those ethnic categories we recorded percentages of physicians
with medical licenses, American board specialty, and specialties with varying percentages of minority or nonminority group physicians, as obtained
from the 1994 medical directory.

Practice locations as shown in the medical directory allowed us to iden-tify those physicians practicing in a state with any one of three levels of African American population as shown in 1990. Of our combined total of 3,787 physicians for whom the medical directory information included a preferred practice location, 35.5 percent ($N = 1,343$) had medical practices in states in the highest tercile of AA population, ranging from 14 percent to 66 percent in the District of Columbia. Another 28.6 percent ($N = 1,084$) practiced in states ranging from 7.4 percent to 14.0 percent Black popula-tion, which is our middle tercile. The remaining 35.9 percent ($N = 1,360$) located their practices in states ranging from 0 percent to 7.4 percent Black population, which is our lowest tercile.

Nearly one-third (32.7 percent; $N = 1,240$) of our total 3,787 physicians practiced in the highest tercile of states in terms of their Hispanic popula-tion, which ranged from 12.2 percent to 39.0 percent Hispanic; 34.2 per-cent ($N = 1,294$) practiced in states in the middle tercile, which ranged from 2.2 percent to 12.2 Hispanic population; and 33.1 percent ($N = 1,253$) practiced in states with the lowest tercile of Hispanic population, ranging from 0 percent to 2.2 percent.

The difference in cutpoints immediately suggests how differently the African American and Hispanic populations are distributed among the var-ious states, a difference that we can also note when we subdivide the His-panic group into Mexican and Puerto Rican fractions, such as the high pro-portion of Mexicans in California and Texas, and the high proportion of Puerto Ricans in New York.

We also could identify practice locations in "big cities" that have large populations of African American or Hispanic populations, or both. For example, an African American city was identified as follows: (1) It is an urban area designated by the Census Bureau as a metropolitan statistical area (either consolidated [CMSA] or primary [PMSA]). The *Statistical Ab-stract* identifies a PMSA as a metropolitan area with a population of one million or more. If an area contains more than one PMSA, it is designated as a CMSA. (2) If a physician practices in a CMSA or PMSA with more than five hundred thousand Blacks, then that practice location was coded as being in an African American city ("1"; otherwise as "0").

Similarly an HI city is so defined if the metropolitan area has more than 500,000 Hispanic Americans.

Geographic regions are defined as in chapter 6 of this book: Northeast, Midwest, West (in which I included Texas), and South.

Practice locations were further characterized by their neighborhoods, as identified by zip code. An AA practice neighborhood was a zip code in which 50 percent or more of the population was Black, and a HI neighborhood had a zip code with greater than 20 percent Hispanic American population. These different cutpoints were selected as being likely to capture the most relevant data.

The income levels of the residents of practice neighborhoods were also easily identified by zip code.

FINDINGS FOR PRACTICE LOCATION

PRACTICE LOCATION BY REGION

How the physicians were distributed in the four regions of the United States that we have defined is shown in table 28. First we see from the column totals that the West is the most common location, with almost 34 percent; followed by the South, 28 percent; with the Northeast and Midwest both attracting close to 20 percent.

All of these findings are in the expected direction, showing that Black physicians are relatively more likely to practice in the South, whereas Hispanic Americans, in particular Mexicans, prefer the West relative to their numbers. Almost 14 percent of the sample practicing in the West were Mexicans, versus almost 2 percent in the other 3 regions.

PRACTICE LOCATION BY STATE

The findings for region suggest that the followed-up physicians tended to locate their practices in states significantly populated by their ethnic groups. Further confirmation of the concentration of minority physicians

TABLE 28. Region of Practice, 1994, by Ethnicity

	NE[a]	MW[b]	W	S	Raw N
% Minority	47.9	45.1	52.0[c]	51.4	864
African American	41.3	41.9	34.9[d]	47.8[e]	537
Hispanic	6.4	2.8	15.5**	2.8[f]	291
% Nonminority	52.1	54.9*	48.0	48.6	1,883
N	706	714	1,265	1,062	3,747
%	18.8	19.1	33.8	28.3	100.0

[a]No significant differences found.
[b]Significant nonminority preference
[c]$p < .05$, but with relatively fewer African American.
[d]$p < .00005$ and relatively more Hispanic.
[e]Significantly more African American but with fewer Hispanic ($p < .00005$).
[f]Fewer Hispanic in the South than expected by chance ($p = .00005$ compared to all others).
*$p < .05$.   **$p < .00005$.

in states with the highest proportion of their minority groups is found in tables 29 and 30.

Minority physicians had a significant tendency to establish their practice in states with the highest third of their minority group population, as defined above, detailed in tables 29 and 30. This finding was true for both male and female minority physicians. Almost 43 percent of African American male physicians established their practices in the highest third of states grouped by percentage Black population, compared to almost 30 percent of nonminority male physicians. The corresponding statistics for female physicians were 47 percent African American and 30.3 percent nonminority.

Nearly 67 percent of Hispanic male physicians established their practices in the highest third of states grouped by percentage of Hispanic population, compared to 29 percent of nonminority male physicians; for females the corresponding percentages were almost 68 percent Hispanic and about 33 percent nonminority.

With respect to sample physicians establishing practices in states having the highest tercile of African American population, specific findings for the ethnic groups were as shown in table 31.

TABLE 29. Practice Location of Black and Nonminority Physicians, by Proportion of Black Population in State

Proportion of Black Population in State	Black Physicians	Nonminority Physicians
Lowest tercile	28.5 −	41.0 +
Middle tercile	27.7	29.3
Highest tercile	43.7 +	29.7 −
Total	99.9[a]	100.0

Note: p of $\chi^2 < .000005$. A plus sign indicates more than expected by chance alone. A minus sign indicates fewer than expected by chance alone.

[a]Does not total 100% because of rounding.

TABLE 30. Practice Location of Hispanic and Nonminority Physicians, by Proportion of Hispanic Population in State

Proportion of Hispanic Population in State	Hispanic Physicians	Nonminority Physicians
Lowest tercile	12.6 −	34.8 +
Middle tercile	20.3 −	35.4 +
Highest tercile	67.1 +	29.8 −

Note: p of $\chi^2 < .000005$. A plus sign indicates more than expected by chance alone. A minus sign indicates fewer than expected by chance alone.

Among all the groups of physicians, only Blacks chose to establish practices in states with the highest proportions of Blacks in their populations. For Mexicans the findings were the reverse of those for Blacks, whereas those for Native Americans and for Puerto Ricans were not substantially different than those for nonminority physicians. Despite some small sample sizes, the findings are stable and reliable, as indication that only Black physicians chose, in disproportionately large numbers, to establish their practices in states with high proportions of Black population.

For states with the highest level of Hispanic population (the highest tercile), specific findings for the ethnic groups were as follows (see table 32): A high concentration of Mexican physicians followed the Hispanic population, and also a disproportionately high proportion of Puerto Rican physicians. Nonminority physicians were disproportionately absent from high-Hispanic states, whereas Blacks and Native Americans were present in proportionate numbers.

In conclusion, the findings of high concentrations of African American physicians in high African American states, and of Mexican and Puerto Rican physicians in high Hispanic states, sharply contrasted with the relative absence of nonminority physicians from those states.

TABLE 31. Ethnicity of Physicians Who Established Practice in States in Highest Tercile of Black Population

	N	n	%
African American	1,550	678	43.7 +
Mexican American	221	23	10.4 −
Puerto Rican	76	25	32.9
Native American	26	7	26.9
Nonminority	1,901	607	31.9 −

Note: p of χ^2 < .000005. A plus sign indicates more than expected by chance alone. A minus sign indicates fewer than expected b chance alone.

TABLE 32. Ethnicity of Physicians Who Established Practice in States in Highest Tercile of Hispanic Population

	N	n	%
African American	1,550	511	33.0
Mexican American	221	167	75.6 +
Puerto Rican	76	34	44.7 +
Native American	26	11	42.3
Nonminority	1,901	514	27.0 −

Note: p of χ^2 < .000005. A plus sign indicates more than expected by chance alone. A minus sign indicates fewer than expected by chance alone.

PRACTICE LOCATION BY CITIES

We further honed the characterization of the areas in which followed-up physicians established their practices, by focusing on those physicians who established their practices in cities with populations of more than half a million African American or Hispanic residents.

An analysis of practice locations in big cities with more than five hundred thousand African American population shows the following (see table 33): African American physicians located their practices in cities with large populations of their group. Other minority group members did not have a significant tendency to locate in cities with high African American populations. Comparing both Hispanic populations together (Mexican American and Puerto Rican), there are some cities with a high frequency of both Hispanic and African American population. The high correlation coefficient of 0.69 indicates that 592 out of 3,788 physicians (15.6 percent) located in cities high in both minority populations, whereas 427 (11.3 percent) located in cities high in one or the other, and 2,769 (73.1 percent) located in cities that did not have significant critical masses of either.

The corresponding trends for practice location in a high-Hispanic city are shown in table 34. Hispanic physicians significantly tended to locate in

TABLE 33. Physicians Who Established Practice in Cities with High Black Population, by Ethnicity and Gender

	%	N
Minority	33.3 +	1,887
Men	31.3 +	1,513
Women	41.2 +	357
Nonminority	17.1	1,901
Men	16.6	1,652
Women	19.4	222
African American	36.2 +	1,550
Men	34.3 +	1,226
Women	43.5 +	310
Native American	11.5[a]	26
Mexican American	19.9[a]	221
Puerto Rican	22.4[a]	76

Note: p of $\chi^2 < .000005$. Gender-specific frequencies do not total to the group frequencies due to cases with missing data for gender. A plus sign indicates more than expected by chance alone. A minus sign indicates fewer than expected by chance alone.

[a]Not significant.

cities high in concentrations of their groups, and African American physicians were also practicing in those areas, which may simultaneously be high in African American population. Nonminority physicians were significantly less likely to locate in areas high in minority group population.

PRACTICE LOCATION BY NEIGHBORHOODS

We broke down the practice location preferences of followed-up physicians in table 35 to the level of practice neighborhoods, indicated by the zip code of the preferred practice location. This made these trends even more evident.

Quite clearly African American physicians established their practices in high African American neighborhoods (zip codes with more than 50 percent African American population). No others, including other minorities, select those areas.

We looked at predominantly Hispanic practice neighborhoods, defined as zip codes with more than 20 percent Hispanic population (see table 36). Clearly Hispanic physicians followed their populations, but there was also a strong trend for African American physicians to practice in those neighborhoods.

PRACTICE LOCATION BY AREA INCOME

For the purposes of this study we defined a "low-income area" as one in which the average household income is less than $15,000 according to census data; "middle income areas" have incomes greater than $25,000 annually; and "high income areas" have incomes exceeding $50,000 for an average household. These cutpoints are used by the Census Bureau. A total

TABLE 34. Ethnicity of Physicians Who Established Practice in Cities with High Hispanic Population

	%	N
Hispanic	23.6 +	301
Mexican American	24.4 +	221
Puerto Rican	21.1 +	76
African American	21.5 +	1,550
Nonminority	13.1 −	1,901

Note: p of χ^2 < .000005. Gender-specific frequencies do not total to the group frequencies due to cases with missing data for gender. A plus sign indicates more than expected by chance alone. A minus sign indicates fewer than expected by chance alone.

TABLE 35. Physicians Who Practice in Neighborhoods with More Than 50 Percent Black Population, by Ethnicity and Gender

	%	N
Minorities	24.4 +	1,708
Males	23.7 +	1,371
Females	26.2 +	321
Nonminorities	6.6 −	1,748
Males	6.4 −	1,519
Females	8.9 −	203
African American	28.5 +	1,413
Hispanic	4.6 −	262
Mexican American	5.5 −	199
Puerto Rican	1.6 −	61

Note: p of $\chi^2 < .000005$. Gender-specific frequencies do not total to the group frequencies due to cases with missing data for gender. A plus sign indicates more than expected by chance alone. A minus sign indicates fewer than expected by chance alone.

TABLE 36. Physicians Who Practice in Neighborhoods with More Than 20 Percent Hispanic Population, by Ethnicity and Gender

	%	N
Minorities	18.5 +**	1,708
Males	18.3 +*	1,371
Females	19.6 −*	321
Nonminorities	6.9−	1,748
Males	6.9 −	1,519
Females	5.9 −	203
Hispanic	35.9 +*	262
Mexican American	40.2 +*	199
Puerto Rican	23.0 +*	61
African American	15.1 +*	1,413

Note: Gender-specific frequencies do not total to the group frequencies due to cases with missing data for gender. A plus sign indicates more than expected by chance alone. A minus sign indicates fewer than expected by chance alone.

*p of $\chi^2 < .00005$.   **p of $\chi^2 < .000005$.

of 331 physicians practiced in areas with average household incomes greater than $15,000 and less than $25,000, and so they are not included in some analyses.

For the nation as a whole, 7.1 percent (246 of 3,482) of all minority and nonminority physicians practice in low-income areas; 69.8 percent (2,429 of 3,482) practice in middle-income areas; and 13.7 percent (476 of 3,482) practice in high-income areas. We were unable to completely locate area of practice by income because we lacked zip code data for 8.2 percent (313 of 3,795) of the total physician sample with follow-up data.

We do know which physicians are minority or nonminority: By design the total number of minority physicians was 2,067 or 50 percent of our baseline sample, of 4,134. Therefore, 2,067 nonminority physicians were sampled. Of these 4,134 physicians, 3,795 (91.8 percent) had follow-up data, and 339 (8.2 percent) were lost to follow-up. Of the 3,795 followed-up physicians, 1,889 (49.8 percent) are minority, whereas 1,906 (50.2 percent) are nonminority. It is easily seen that loss to follow-up does not jeopardize the validity of our sampling design.

That only 7.1 percent of this national sample of physicians practice in low-income areas despite the fact that these areas have the greatest need for physician services should not come as a surprise. Our national health care system is essentially based on demand, itself a composite of both the volume of requests for physicians' services *and* the resources to pay for those services. It is responsive to economic market demand rather than health care need. Freedom of choice for physicians to locate according to their preferences or wishes, and freedom of choice for the patients to choose their physicians depending on their ability to pay, are the basic premises on which our health care system operates. Patients who are unable to pay, or who until recent decades were not served because of ethnic or other reasons, were supposedly served by safety-net providers associated with public hospitals or religious charity institutions.

Looking at the nationwide distributions we find that significantly more

TABLE 37. **Income in Area of Practice of Minority and Nonminority Physicians**

	Minority	Nonminority	*N*
Low income	8.3[a]	5.8	246
Middle income	67.9[b]	71.6	2,429
High income	12.8	14.5	476

[a]Minority > nonminority, $p < .005$.
[b]Nonminority > minority, $p < .005$.

minority physicians were practicing in low-income areas and significantly more nonminority physicians were practicing in middle and high income areas (see table 37).

These trends were then subjected to a more complete review by looking at nonminority and minority physicians in the various regions of the nation. What we found is outlined in table 38. Striking differences are noted in this regional analysis: Minority physicians significantly exceeded nonminority physicians in low-income neighborhoods of the Midwest and South by wide margins; nonminority physicians significantly outnumbered minority physicians in middle-income neighborhoods in the Northeast and Midwest; nonminority physicians significantly outnumber minority physicians in high-income neighborhoods in the Northeast. In the West

TABLE 38. Income of Practice Neighborhood, Minority and Nonminority Physicians, by Region

	Minority	Nonminority	Row N
Northeast			
Low income	3.7	4.0	26
Middle income	74.2[a]	81.9	530
High income	18.8[b]	30.3	168
Column N	325	353	678
Column %	52.1	47.9	100
Midwest			
Low income	14.6[c]	6.8	70
Middle income	57.0[d]	73.7	445
High income	10.4	11.8	75
Column N	365	309	674
Column %	54.2	45.8	100
West			
Low income	4.0	3.4	43
Middle income	75.8	71.3	856
High income	11.2	13.2	142
Column N	598	565	1,163
Column %	51.4	48.6	100
South			
Low income	11.3[e]	6.2	83
Middle income	61.8	65.0	598
High income	10.1	9.2	91
Column N	477	466	943
Column %	50.6	49.4	100

[a] = Nonminority > Minority, $p < .05$.
[b] = Nonminority > Minority, $p < .0005$.
[c] = Minority > Nonminority, $p < .005$.
[d] = Nonminority > Minority, $p < .0005$.
[e] = Minority > Nonminority, $p < .01$.

there were no global differences in the distribution of minority and non-minority physicians. (Recall that our definition of the West includes both Texas and California.)

If we zero in on Blacks, the findings are practically identical, since it is the African American physicians whose behavior is reflected in the whole minority group sample. The practice neighborhood pattern for Hispanic physicians (Mexicans and Puerto Ricans) is not clearly distinguishable from nonminority physicians at the regional level of the nation.

PRACTICE LOCATION BY URBAN CONCENTRATIONS OF MINORITY POPULATIONS

We proceeded to look at the practice location choices of followed-up physicians in terms of practicing in an urban area with more than half a million African American residents or more than half a million Hispanic residents.

There were twelve metropolitan areas with more than a half million Black residents. A third of minority group physicians (628 of 1,887) practiced in these areas, compared to 17.1 percent (326 of 1,901) nonminority physicians, of whom practiced in these areas. This predominance of minority group physicians was statistically significant ($p <.000005$), and the differences held true for both male and for female physicians, with a suggested trend that it is even more the case for women than for men: (1) minority male physicians, 31.3 percent, compared with 16.6 percent nonminority; (2) minority female physicians, 41.2 percent, compared with 19.4 percent nonminority female physicians. Relatively more women physicians select these practice locations compared to their male counterparts. As for Blacks only, 36.2 percent of these physicians practiced in these metropolitan areas compared with 17.6 percent of all others ($p < .000005$). Other minorities did not differ significantly from nonminorities: Mexicans, 19.9 percent; Puerto Ricans, 22.4 percent; Native Americans, 11.5 percent; and all nonminority physicians, 17.1 percent.

Our definition of a highly Hispanic metropolitan area was one with more than half a million Hispanic residents. In these nine areas, 21.6 percent of the physicians were minorities, compared with 13.1 percent nonminority. Here again the trend was true for women, with a suggestive trend of women physicians exceeding men in these areas: (1) minority males, 20.5 percent, versus nonminority male, 12.8 percent; (2) minority female physicians, 26.3 percent, versus nonminority females, 14.0 percent.

Hispanic physicians exceeded all others in these metropolitan areas: 23.6 percent (71 of 301) broken down into 24.4 percent (54 of 221) Mexican and 21.1 percent (16 of 76) Puerto Rican. This finding is significant for Hispanic physicians as a whole compared with all others ($p < .005$) and for Mexicans compared to all others ($p < .01$), but not for the Puerto Ricans. It is worth noting that African American physicians contributed 21.5 percent of the physicians to these areas, a contribution that was significantly greater compared with all others combined ($p < .00005$). Three hundred thirty-three of 1,550 Black physicians practiced in such areas versus 323 of 2,233, or 14.5 percent, non-Black. Again this is due to the co-occurrence of high concentrations of Blacks and Hispanics in metropolitan areas like New York or Los Angeles, among others.

As might be expected, these trends are magnified in practice neighborhoods with 50 percent or more Black population. Total minority physicians contributed 24.4 percent of those practicing in such zip codes (416 of 1,708), compared with only 6.6 percent (115 of 1,748) of nonminority physicians, a highly significant finding ($p < .000005$). Again this was true for women as well as men, with women slightly more often practicing in these neighborhoods: (1) minority male 23.7 percent compared with 6.4 percent nonminority male; (2) minority female 26.2 percent compared with 8.9 percent nonminority female.

The great bulk of these physicians were themselves Blacks, 28.5 percent (402 of 1,413) compared with 6.3 percent (128 of 2,039) of all other physicians, a very significant finding ($p < .000005$). Hispanics were no more likely than nonminority physicians to locate in these zip codes: only 4.6 percent did so, including 5.5 percent (11 of 199) of Mexican physicians and 1.6 percent (1 of 61) of Puerto Rican physicians.

We defined significantly Hispanic practice neighborhoods as zip codes with 20 percent or more Hispanic population. Zip codes with high concentrations of Hispanic population tended to not have high concentrations of African American population, as shown by a correlation coefficient of $-.09$ ($p < .000005$) based on the distribution of practice locations in our sample. This gives us a different perspective than in our previous analyses. For example the NY-NNJ-LI CMSA has more than half a million of each group, but the two groups tend to concentrate in different zip codes. Here we find a predominance of minority physicians, 18.5 percent (316 of 1,708) compared with 6.9 percent (121 of 1,748) of nonminority physicians, a highly significant finding ($p < .000005$). This pattern was equally true for male and female physicians, with no suggestive trend that women locate in these areas to a greater extent than men: (1) minority men, 18.3 percent, versus 6.9 percent nonminority; (2) minority female, 19.6 percent, versus nonminority female 5.9 percent.

Here, however, we are able to demonstrate high Hispanic physician preference for these neighborhoods, 35.9 percent (94 of 262) compared with 10.8 percent of all others (343 of 3,190), a very significant finding (p <.000005). Subdividing the Hispanic physicians, Mexicans were present at 40.2 percent (80 of 199) and Puerto Ricans at 23.0 percent (14 of 61), both of which are statistically significant (p < .05). Blacks were present at 15.1 percent (214 of 1,413) in these zip codes, which is significantly greater (p < .0005) than all non-Blacks, who were at 10.9 percent (223 of 2,039).

PRACTICE LOCATION PREFERENCE AND INCOME LEVEL OF THE PHYSICIANS' FAMILY OF ORIGIN

The next important question to answer is how these practice locations relate to the income of the family of origin of the minority physicians. In an earlier chapter we indicated that National Medical Fellowships were the central source of financial aid for minority medical students throughout the 1969–73 period in which these students were in medical school. All minority students accepted into any medical school could apply for financial aid if they so desired. We therefore were able to stratify our minority physicians into three categories based on their medical school NMF application status. We know further that those who applied for financial aid and received it had average family incomes in 1970 dollars of $8,880; those who were rejected had average family incomes of $14,960. Those who never applied had family incomes of unknown amounts, but we surmised that they assumed they were ineligible or did not wish to apply for other reasons. Remember also that all of our minority sample consisted of medical school applicants who identified themselves as minority members on their medical school application in order to be identified as such by the Association of American Medical Colleges publication sent to all medical school admissions offices.

Considerable comment has been made on whether affirmative action programs should address all minority applicants or only to those who are economically disadvantaged. We are defining those who applied for and received an NMF award as being the most economically disadvantaged because of their extremely low average family income. Even those rejected because of relatively higher average family incomes were predominantly from impoverished family backgrounds.

When we examined the choice of physicians to practice in metropolitan areas with more than half a million African American residents (see table 39), we saw that NMF applicants were likely to set up practices in these urban areas at about double the rate for nonminority physicians. This was true whether NMF applications came from backgrounds of very low family income (recipients, average $8,800) or relatively higher family incomes (rejectees, average $14,960). There was in fact a trend suggesting that relatively better off African Americans more often selected these areas compared to their less economically favorable peers. Both of these groups of minority applicants came from families much less favored than nonminorities, whose average family income was probably almost twice as high.

When we examined the choice of physicians to practice in metropolitan areas with more than half a million Hispanic residents (see table 40), we saw that NMF recipients also significantly preferred these areas, and again the relatively better off NMF applicants (i.e., rejectees) chose these areas even more than those who had lower family incomes (i.e., recipients).

These findings do not support those who maintain that affirmative action programs should only be aimed at the most economically disadvantaged among the minority groups.

TABLE 39. Frequency of Practice in Metropolitan Area with More Than 500,000 Blacks

| Practice in Metropolitan Area with More Than 500,000 Blacks | Minority, by NMF Grant Status | | | | |
	Nonminority	Never Applied	Rejected	Received	Total N
No	82.8%	71.9%	59.6%	66.7%	2,805
Yes	17.2%	28.1%	40.4%[a]	33.3%[b]	904
N	1,096	306	265	1,272	3,749

Note: p of $\chi^2 < .000005$.
[a]Rejectees > nonminority.
[b]Received > nonminority.

TABLE 40. Frequency of Practice in Metropolitan Area with More Than 500,000 Hispanics

| Practice in Metropolitan Area with More Than 500,000 Hispanics | Minority, by NMF Grant Status | | | | |
	Nonminority	Never Applied	Rejected	Received	Total N
No	86.8%	82.0%	74.0%	66.7%	3,097
Yes	13.2%	18.0%	26.0%[a]	21.8%[b]	652
N	1,906	306	265	1,272	3,749

Note: p of $\chi^2 < .000005$.
[a]Rejectees > nonminority.
[b]Received > nonminority.

FINDINGS FOR MINORITY AND NONMINORITY PHYSICIAN CHARACTERISTICS

LICENSURE

Significantly fewer minority physicians were licensed compared with their nonminority peers, minorities 92.9 percent (1,754 of 1,888) versus nonminority 94.5 percent (1,797 of 1,900), a difference that although small was statistically significant ($p < .05$). A slightly higher percentage of males in each group were licensed compared with females: (1) minority males, 93.3 percent, and females, 91.3 percent; (2) nonminority males, 94.7 percent, and females, 93.2 percent. The lower rate of licensure among the minority group physicians is produced primarily by the African American subgroup, which accounts for 83 percent of the minority group of physicians. Of the Black physicians, 92.3 percent were licensed (1,432 of 1,551). This rate was significantly ($p < .05$) lower than that of the Mexicans 96.4 percent (213 of 221), but not significantly different than those of either the Puerto Ricans 93.4 percent (71 of 76) or the Native Americans 92.3 percent (24 of 26).

ATTAINMENT OF A SPECIALTY BOARD CERTIFICATION

Significantly fewer minority graduates became board-certified specialists compared with their nonminority peers ($p < .00005$): 61.1 percent of minorities (1,154 of 1,889) versus 89.4 percent for nonminorities (1,701 of 1,902).

Here again within each group more men than women had received certification: (1) minority men, 61.1 percent (926 of 1,515), versus minority women, 59.9 percent (214 of 357), which is not a statistically significant difference; (2) nonminority men, 88.7 percent (1,490 of 1,653), versus nonminority women, 85.6 percent, a statistically significant difference ($p < .05$).

From findings reported in chapter 6 we know that almost 100 percent of both minority and nonminority groups entered residency training programs for specialist training. We do not know how many dropped out before completing the required three or four years of training. We know that many young physicians who complete residency training and become "board eligible" do not take the board examination; others take the examination and fail. Our data do not clarify these issues.

Similarly too the pattern of having specialty certification within minority groups showed the lowest percentage usually for African Americans 59.7 percent (926 of 1,532), significantly lower than the percentage of Mexicans 68.8 percent (152 of 221) ($p < .01$); but not statistically different than the percentages of Puerto Ricans 67.1 percent (51 of 76) or Native Americans 57.7 percent (15 of 26). Again nonminorities had the largest percentage, 89.4 percent (1,701 of 1,902) ($p < .000005$).

When we look at whether minority group physicians classified by their NMF status were more or less likely to become certified specialists, we see that there were no statistically significant differences among those who never applied, 64.4 percent (197 of 306), rejectees, 63.4 percent (168 of 265), and recipients, 59.9 percent (762 of 1,273).

African American graduates of the traditionally Black medical schools, Meharry and Howard, were less likely to become certified specialists than African American graduates from other medical schools. Of the Black graduates of Meharry and Howard, 48.5 percent had become certified specialists (115 of 237) versus 61.6 percent of all other African American graduates (808 of 1,312), a very significant difference ($p < .0005$).

This difference becomes even more pronounced when all minority group graduates of Meharry and Howard are compared with all other minority group physicians. Of the minority graduates of Meharry and Howard, 48.5 percent became certified specialists (117 of 241), compared with all other minority physicians 62.9 percent (1,032 of 1,642), a very significant difference ($p < .0005$).

We then turned to minority graduates of medical schools other than Meharry and Howard to see if having graduated from one of the ten private medical schools (other than Meharry and Howard) that produced the most minority graduates, or from one of the ten public medical schools that produced the most minority graduates, predicted becoming a certified specialist. We found that 65.5 percent of those who graduated from the private medical schools became certified specialists (230 of 351), not significantly more than the percentage of other minority graduates, 62.2 percent (806 of 1,296). We also found that 64.4 percent of those who graduated from one of the public schools that produced the most minority graduates became certified specialists (250 of 388), which was not significantly more than the 62.4 percent of other minority graduates (786 of 1,259) who became specialists.

ATTAINMENT OF MORE THAN ONE BOARD CERTIFICATION

Among physicians with certification by at least one specialty board, minority physicians were less likely to be boarded in a second specialty, 6.8 percent (78 of 1,154), than were nonminority physicians, 8.8 percent

(150 of 1,701), a difference barely missing statistical significance ($p =$ .0547).

Differences between males and females, while present, were smaller and not significant: (1) minority men, 6.7 percent (62 of 926), versus minority women, 6.5 percent (14 of 214); (2) nonminority men, 8.9 percent (133 of 1,490), versus nonminority women, 7.4 percent (14 of 190).

Within the minority group of physicians, ethnic group differences were also less frequent and not significant, although still showing a suggestive trend: Blacks, 6.7 percent (62 of 926), Mexicans, 8.6 percent (13 of 152), Puerto Ricans, 2.0 percent (1 of 51), and Native Americans, 6.7 percent (1 of 15).

COMPARING MINORITY AND NONMINORITY BOARD SPECIALISTS

In this section we compare the 1,154 minority physicians who are board certified with the 1,701 nonminority physician specialists. To give the analysis a simple presentation, the discussion is limited to the major specialties: internal medicine, family practice, surgery, obstetrics-gynecology, pediatrics, and psychiatry.

Table 41 illustrates that for all physicians who have become certified, similar percentages of minority and nonminority physicians chose internal medicine, family practice, surgery, and psychiatry. A statistically significantly higher percentage of minority physicians than nonminority physicians selected obstetrics-gynecology (OB-GYN) and pediatrics.

As shown in table 42, nearly twice as many minority men compared with nonminority men chose obstetrics-gynecology, whereas there was no such trend among women. Among minority women the preference for pediatrics is twice that of nonminority women.

From the observations delineated in table 43 we conclude that African Americans chose family practice less often than expected by chance, and both OB-GYN and pediatrics more often than expected. Mexicans and Native Americans chose family practice significantly more often than all

TABLE 41. Specialties of Minority and Nonminority Physicians

	Internal Medicine	Family Practice	Surgery	OB-GYN	Pediatrics	Psychiatry	N
Minority	28.0%	14.0%	5.7%	10.9%	13.3%	4.8%	1,154
Nonminority	28.5%	13.2%	6.8%	6.2%[a]	9.5%[b]	4.9%	1,701

[a] p of $\chi^2 < .00005$.
[b] p of $\chi^2 < .005$.

other physicians. Puerto Ricans chose family practice 6.4 points more often than the nonminority physicians, although the result is not statistically significant.

Our other findings on specialty differences are as follows: Minority physicians are present in statistically greater frequency in obstetrics and gynecology and in pediatrics. The numbers of nonminority physicians are significantly greater in allergy, emergency medicine, neurology, orthopedic surgery, pathology, and radiology. Both groups are equally represented in internal medicine, colorectal surgery, dermatology, family practice, genetics, neurosurgery, nuclear medicine, ophthalmology, physical medicine and rehabilitation, plastic surgery, urology, and psychiatry. Our samples were of sufficient size to indicate that these differences were not due to chance and were significant in all instances with a probability of less than .05 that the event occurred by chance.

TABLE 42. Specialties of Minority and Nonminority Physicians, by Gender

	Internal Medicine (%)	Family Practice (%)	Surgery (%)	OB-GYN (%)	Pediatrics (%)	Psychiatry (%)	N
Male							
Minority	30.0	14.0	6.5	11.3	9.0	4.4	926
Nonminority	28.6	14.0	7.0	5.6[a]	8.6	4.4	1,490
Female							
Minority	19.6	13.6	2.3	8.9	31.3	6.5	214
Nonminority	27.9	7.9	5.8	10.5	15.8[b]	8.4	190

[a] p of $\chi^2 < .00005$.
[b] p of $\chi^2 < .005$.

TABLE 43. Percentage of Various Specialties among Minority and Nonminority Physicians, by Ethnicity

	Internal Medicine ($N = 808$)	Family Practice ($N = 385$)	Surgery ($N = 182$)	OB-GYN ($N = 231$)	Pediatrics ($N = 314$)	Psychiatry ($N = 138$)	N
African American	28.1	11.3 −	6.3	12.3	13.5	4.9	926
Mexican American	26.3	25.0 +	4.6	6.6	11.2	3.3	152
Puerto Rican	35.3	19.6	0	3.9	19.6 +	7.8	51
Native American	20.0	40.0 +	6.7	0	0	6.7	15
Other minority	33.3	16.7	0	0	0	6.7	6
Nonminority	28.5	13.2	6.8	6.2	9.5 −	4.9	1,701
							2,851

Note: A plus sign indicates more than expected by chance alone. A minus sign indicates fewer than expected by chance alone.

HAS AFFIRMATIVE ACTION WORKED?

Affirmative action programs in medicine have had a tremendous impact, have improved the quality of health care in minority communities, and have made a major head start in equalizing the medical education and training for minority professionals. As recently as 1970 Blacks made up only 2.8 percent (or 1,042) of the 37,690 enrolled medical students. By 1977 Blacks comprised 6.0 percent (or 3,587) of the 60,039 total medical school enrollment. There were only about 100 board-certified specialists who were Black among the 4,000 physicians, of whom 85 percent had graduated from either Howard or Meharry, the two traditional Black medical schools. Our sample of 1,889 minority graduates includes 1,552 Blacks who graduated in the years 1973–77, and who were followed-up in the year 1994. From the data presented in this chapter we can report that 1,150 minority graduates have become certified in at least one medical specialty, including 926 African American graduates and 224 other minority graduates; as well as 1,701 nonminority graduates. In our followed-up sample of 1,884 minority physicians, 7.1 percent graduated from Meharry and 6.1 percent from Howard, so that these two traditionally African American medical schools contributed only 13.2 percent of the minority students who graduated in the five-year period 1973–77. All other medical schools were now producing minority graduates, more than 85 percent of minority physicians, a complete reversal from an earlier decade. The reader should bear in mind that our baseline sample of 2,067 minority medical school graduates is only a sample, representing 45.7 percent of the 4,370 minority graduates in that time period. The baseline sample of 2,067 nonminority graduates represented a 3.4 percent sample of the 61,518 medical school graduates of that group during the same five-year period.

The social benefits of these affirmative action programs is the issue of relevant concern. Are there benefits both to the minority communities and the nation as a whole? We believe we have shown startling gains, which can be explained as follows. These young minority physicians are meeting the urgent unmet medical needs of underserved minority communities, going into areas avoided by others, often into locations offering fewer financial benefits or status gains.

WILL THEY RETURN TO THE GHETTO?

In *Blacks, Medical School, and Society* (1971, 147–63), I devoted a chapter to this question that was and is commonly raised in debates over affirmative action as a valuable social policy. It was my position then, as now, that providing first-class medical educational opportunity to greater numbers of qualified Blacks and other underrepresented minorities would result in improved health care in underserved communities since most minority physicians, especially Blacks, primarily treat Black patients. This is a consequence of racially segregated neighborhoods, in both the inner city and the suburbs, where both Black physicians and their patients live. Even though Black physicians have greater freedom in selecting the neighborhood in which they work and live, only a small minority would voluntarily choose both a practice location and a place to live far removed from their social support network. Without giving it conscious thought, most Black physicians realize that to build a practice, they need the help of family and relatives, friends, neighbors, the local church, and their Black colleagues who are physicians or other professionals. From my personal observations of Black physicians over a period of fifty years, less than 5 percent choose to avoid Black patients who would be referred to them. Even if the Black sets up an office in the downtown area, or a professional office building outside the Black community, he will usually have a predominantly Black patient caseload.

Black and White people in the United States have up until the present time lived in separate worlds, with separate histories from the era of slavery to the present time. Racially segregated housing and neighborhoods have served to isolate Blacks from mainstream American social, economic, and political opportunity, and left them with a burden of physical, psychological, and behavioral impairment thwarting their full developmental potential. Massey and Denton (1993) describe this national scourge that cripples all of our major metropolitan areas in *American Apartheid: Segregation and the Making of the Underclass*.

We have shown convincingly that minority physicians graduating from medical schools during the 1970s are tending to establish their practices in relatively low-income neighborhoods where their minority groups tend to live, bringing many new resources of medical care to these frequently blighted communities. A parallel demonstration has been made to show that their nonminority peers graduating in the same time period are predictably establishing their practices in predominantly White middle class communities, their communities of origin. For both groups it is our surmise that they are demonstrating the sociological determinants of professional behavior, the pressure of group conformity that is usually strong enough to override an individual's conscious choice. But if it is true that young professionals will tend to follow their own support groups, does this not give us another vantage point from which to answer the question: "Will they return to the ghetto?" In large measure both minority and nonminority physicians return to their respective ghettoes. Not only does this speak strongly for the necessity of creating an American professional class that reflects our national diversity, but it underscores the fact that there is considerable unfinished business in producing physicians who will without coercion freely choose to serve all the people, rich as well as poor; rural as well as urban; North, South, East, and West. In an earlier chapter I mentioned the strong plea by Fitzhugh Mullan, who decries the fact that American medical schools still graduate only about half the physicians required to fill the residency training positions offered by our hospitals. Having done so for half a century we have by now traditionally become dependent on the importation of foreign medical graduates while we refuse to admit more than half of the very able young Americans who apply to our medical schools each year (Mullan 2000). This may be one example of challenges we face in our aspiration to bring more equitable human services and not just medical services, to the American public, because of our reluctance to rely on strong national planning rather than free market choices.

History is the record of changes in social group behavior, and it reveals the predictable tendency of empowered groups to pass on their dominance to their children and thereby protect their vested interests. This history repeats itself until accidental developments present a crisis requiring a loosening up of the social hierarchy, particularly in a relatively open political society. Earlier chapters have traced the course of changes in the past fifty years: the field of medicine is no longer the exclusive preserve of White Protestant males from the middle class serving primarily its own interests but has opened up sequentially to Catholics; Jews; foreign medical graduats; women; Asians; and members of underrepresented ethnic minority groups, including Black Americans, changes that hold the promise of improving the health and life outcomes of all our citizens.

THE IMPACT OF AFFIRMATIVE ACTION IN MEDICAL SCHOOLS: PREVIOUS STUDIES

Keith, Bell, and Williams (1987) with support of the Association of American Medical College database followed the developing career pattern of the graduating class of 1975 up to 1982. The 714 minority graduates, a total sample, were compared with 1,862, or a 20 percent sample, of their nonminority classmates. Survey questionnaire data and American Medical Association physician profile information were used to measure outcomes. Their findings were, as confirmed in our study, that minority physicians were more often in primary care practices and were located twice as often in underserved neighborhoods with significantly more Medicaid patients. These were considered to be positive outcomes of affirmative action. Also, while only 6.3 percent of the 1975 graduates were members of minority groups, this represented only one-half of the 12 percent target that the AAMC had set in 1970. Nonetheless, the number of minority graduates were several times the number or percentage of minority graduates in the decades before affirmative action.

Shortfalls of affirmative action, as perceived by Keith and colleagues, were the finding that only about 50 percent of the minority group were board certified in any field compared with 75 percent of the nonminority group. There seemed to be uncertainty as to whether or not it should be considered a positive outcome if these young minority physicians were in medical research or academic medicine, or were practicing in a predominantly nonminority community. Black patients constituted 56 percent of the patient population of the Black graduates, while all other physicians had only 8 to 14 percent Black patients. There was uncertainty about what might be considered the ideal proportion of Black patients who should have been on the caseload of the Black physicians. In other words, the integration of minority physicians in a profile of practice similar to all American physicians may have been considered incompatible with the aim of increasing access to better medical care for underserved minority communities.

In my view, these uncertainties reflect a fundamental confusion about the aims of affirmative action. As I mentioned in 1971 (162), our aim should be to provide a superior educational experience for minority and nonminority physicians. A racially and ethnically diverse learning experience would improve the future health care for the entire American community. Specifically, young Black physicians should not be required or encouraged to work only with Black patients. Black and White physicians should be comfortably competent in working with Black or White patients. From my personal experience and observations of colleagues, a Black physician who has a racially integrated circle of professional associates and friends will automatically have a racially integrated practice. An integrated education and training experience make this more likely, but it is not a common finding. Young Black physicians should be encouraged to exercise the same freedom of choice given all young physicians to enter any branch of medicine including all areas of specialty and all areas of teaching, research, clinical practice, or administration. A color-blind society is in my opinion the ultimate ideal: "With increasing desegregation in many areas of American life, and an increasing receptivity to a racially integrated society, it is most unlikely that Black and White health care systems and markets can be maintained, even if racist extremists attempt to keep these segregated systems artificially intact" (Curtis 1971, 162–63).

The story of Dr. Ben Carson illustrates this point (Carson 1990). He was raised in inner-city Detroit by a mother with a third-grade education who nonetheless inspired Ben and his older brother Curtis to become academic achievers. Both he and his brother, now an engineer, were below-average students headed nowhere, but at a certain point of time their mother insisted on their becoming regular visitors to the library and that they read two books a week. Surprisingly, after accepting this challenge a new world opened up for them (he was in the fifth grade at the time). By the time he was in the seventh grade he was the top student in his class. He won a scholarship to Yale in 1969, from which he graduated in 1973. He was accepted at the University of Michigan School of Medicine, graduating in 1977. He was one of the 2 out of 175 applicants accepted to Johns Hopkins neurosurgery residency program, which he completed in 1982. The following year he was made director of pediatric neurosurgery, a position he still holds, and he is an associate professor at the Johns Hopkins Medical School. Patients from all over the world seek him out because he has performed some of the most difficult and highly publicized successful operations on children. His professional career is certainly a fulfillment of affirmative action in medicine. He serves as an inspirational model not only for Black youngsters but all who struggle against great odds to fulfill their potential despite being born into extreme social and economic disadvantage.

Racially segregated neighborhoods are still the rule; it would require a high level of national, political, economic, and social leadership commitment to open up the national housing market and bring it to an end. Massey and Denton (1993) suggest ways this might be done, but as Nathan Glazer (1993), pointed out in his review of this impressive argument, "Massive redistribution of persons in our nation's ghettos would require government action on a scale that is simply not possible in a democracy." Given the fact that indices of segregation have grown or remained essentially intact in recent decades, and straightforward support of racial integration has given way to increased ethnic territoriality and polarization on both sides of the racial divide, no immediate end of ghetto communities seems to be in sight.

Given this state of affairs, it is encouraging to document the contribution to an improved society that can be made by affirmative action programs. Studies by Keith et al. (1987) and by Cantor et al. (1996) confirm our findings that minority physicians are bringing improved health care to minority people wherever they live. Cantor et al. made telephone surveys of large samples of minority and nonminority young physicians in 1987 and in 1991. In 1987 a sample of 2,344 was interviewed both in 1987 and in 1991;

another 2,237 were interviewed in 1991 only. Findings clearly demonstrated that minority physicians were several times more likely to serve minority, poor, and Medicaid patients, and this practice pattern was stable over the four-year period. Significantly more women served underserved populations. There were indications that, controlling for race and ethnicity, physicians from lower socioeconomic backgrounds more often served underserved communities. However, this was a weaker association than race. They concluded that substituting socioeconomic disadvantage for minority group status in affirmative action programs would seriously impair levels of service currently delivered to minority group communities.

Our findings are also similar to those reported by Komaromy et al. (1996), who surveyed 718 primary care physicians from fifty-one California counties in 1993 to examine the relationship between physician's race or ethnicity and characteristics of the patients they served. They found that communities with high proportions of Black and Hispanic residents were four times as likely as others to have a shortage of physicians, regardless of community income. Black physicians practiced in areas where the percentage of Black residents was nearly five times as high, on average, as in areas where other physicians practice. Hispanic physicians practiced in areas where the percentage of other Hispanic residents was twice as high as areas where other physicians practiced. Black physicians cared for significantly more patients whose insurance coverage was Medicaid, and Hispanic physicians treated more patients who were uninsured. The authors commented that dismantling affirmative action programs "may threaten health care for both poor people and members of minority groups in California." The findings were based on a random sample of 1,008 physicians who were surveyed, and the response rate was 71 percent: the physicians were 5 percent Black, 6 percent Hispanic, 1.6 percent Asian, and 73 percent White. Our data do not rely on survey responses but rather are taken completely from the AMA physician directory for 1994 and census data, as documented.

Moy and Bartman (1995) analyzed data from the 1987 National Medical Expenditure Survey to examine the relationship between physicians' race and the care of racial minority and medically indigent patients. All survey respondents were over eighteen years old and identified a specific physician as their usual source of care. This was a sample of 15,081, corresponding to a population estimate of 116 million Americans. Findings were that 14.4 percent identified a non-White physician as their main source of care; minority patients were more than four times more likely to receive care from a non-White physician than were non-Hispanic White patients. Low-income, Medicaid, and uninsured patients also were more than four times more likely to receive care from a non-White physician than were non-Hispanic White patients. Low-income, Medicaid, and uninsured patients also were more likely served by minority physicians.

Minority physicians also treated patients who reported worse health, more emergency room visits, more hospitalizations, more acute or chronic complaints, more functional limitations and psychological symptoms, as well as longer visits. Moy and Bartman point out that non-White physicians are therefore particularly vulnerable to being financially penalized by caring for such patients, who, along with their doctors, would be avoided by capitation medical care arrangements. In that study there were 2,446 non-White physicians, and 12,685 White physicians. Patients of the two largest non-White physician groups, 648 Blacks and 926 Asians, were examined separately.

Moy and Bartman mention that AAMC surveys of medical school graduates report that minority physicians reported disproportionate plans to serve their own group but not other minority groups. In contrast, their study demonstrated that "both Black and Asian physicians were more likely to care for minority patients outside their own minority group" (1517). Controlling for physician sex, specialization, workplace, and geographic location did not affect their findings. Their study could not identify the reasons why non-White physicians are more likely to care for minority, medically indigent, and sicker patients. Because we have no survey or interview data in our study, we also are unable to determine the motivations for practice locations of our samples, but we present the bare facts that our minority physicians tended to practice in underserved areas.

The question would arise as to whether or not a race-neutral medical school admissions policy might not produce graduates who would tend also to practice in underserved areas. Candidates for medical school admission might be selected because their slightly lower than average grade point averages and test scores might reflect adverse life circumstances.

One study shows that a race-neutral affirmative action program produces a quite different outcome. During the twenty-year period 1968 to 1987 the University of California at Davis admitted 20 percent of its students, a total of 356, as special consideration admissions. Special admissions were defined as a race-neutral group that included students with less than a GPA of 3.0 (4.0 scale) and/or an MCAT average score less than 10 for the four test subscores; this group was matched with students admitted under regular admission criteria.

The special group contained 33 percent who did not meet the minimum GPA for regular admissions, 44 percent who did not meet minimum MCAT scores, and 23 percent who met neither. In background the special admission students were 35 percent women; 46 percent non-Hispanic Whites; 42.7 percent underrepresented minority groups in categories of Black, Native American, Mexican American, mainland Puerto Rican; and 11 percent Asian and minority groups not included in the previous categories. Among the regularly admitted students, only 4.0 percent were underrepresented minority students. Graduation rates were the same for special admission and other students, nor was there a difference in their postgraduate training choices, their specialty certification status, or their description of patients served. This indicates that race-neutral affirmative action based on lower GPA and/or MCAT scores does not predict future specialty or medical practice experience (Davidson and Lewis 1997).

DEMOGRAPHIC DIFFERENCES OF OTHER BLACK PATIENTS

The Census Bureau released statistics on Blacks and Whites comparing households in February 2000 to coincide with Black History Month (more complete statistics on this topic were made available on the Census Bureau's website <www.census.org>). Some of these findings provide a valuable frame of reference in understanding social gains that Black physicians are contributing to their people and to the nation. Many more Black households are headed by a woman without a partner living at home. Married couples head 47 percent of the 8.4 million Black households, 45 percent or 3.8 million are led by a lone woman, versus a similar situation for 13.0 percent of the nation's 53.1 million White households.

Overall the Black population is also younger: 33 percent of the 35 million Blacks are age eighteen or younger, compared with 24 percent of American's 193 million Whites. It is anticipated that the Black population will rise to be 59.2 million in the year 2050, a 70 percent increase, at which time the Black share of the total population would have increased slightly from 13 percent to 15 percent. In education, 77 percent of Blacks age twenty-five and over had completed a high school education, while 15 percent had bachelor's degrees. Among comparable Whites, high school graduates are 88 percent, and 28 percent have a college degree or higher. More than 55 percent of Blacks live in the South, and more than 86 percent live in cities or surrounding suburbs (i.e., metropolitan areas), both more than is the case for Whites. Our findings on the geographical distribution of minority versus nonminority physicians show that the minority physicians are making valiant efforts to meet the health care needs of their people, and that even specialty choices such as the high prevalence of specialists in OB-GYN and in pediatrics mirror these health care needs.

Freeman and Payne, in an editorial in the *New England Journal of Medicine* (2000), called attention to the "growing body of compelling and disturbing evidence" pointing to inferior health care for Black Americans, "even if they are on equal economic footing with Whites." Differences both in access to treatment and quality of care are "at least part of the reason why the rates of death from some diseases are higher among Blacks than among Whites." Particular attention is called to the fact that Black and Hispanic patients with severe pain are not able to obtain adequate pain relief because pharmacists in minority communities do not stock standard supplies of opiate medications. Why do they not supply these medications? Because they believe that opiate addicts abound in these neighborhoods, that they will be burglarized and ripped off by addicts desperate to obtain drugs, and that it is simply safer not to have opiates in stock. The end result is that the vast majority of the minority community cannot find a drugstore that stocks opiate painkillers prescribed by their physicians. This is a medical version of racial profiling, which is even more lethal in its consequences for patients suffering from a terminal illness like cancer that often causes unimaginable misery and pain. Blacks have a higher-than-average incidence of cancer, and higher rates of death from cancer than any other ethnic group.

The problem goes far beyond terminal cancer. As Freeman and Payne point out, pain that is a sequel to bone fracture or to postoperative surgery of any kind results in the same kind of medical racial neglect.

Lower cancer survival rates for Blacks compared with Whites results from the fact that Whites are treated in earlier stages of their illness, when it is more curable, a finding that stands despite income parity between Whites and Blacks, or even without regard to their insurance coverage, or access to care. Even Blacks who need renal transplants for chronic kidney failure receive such organ transplants less often than Whites—again without respect to income. In the presence of life-threatening coronary artery disease, diagnostic evaluations for symptoms indicating the need for bypass surgery are less often completed for Blacks than for Whites of comparable economic class. It is a common thread, Freeman and Payne conclude, that "physicians, as well as pharmacists, police officers, and others, must learn to see people not through the lens of race but instead as the individual persons they are." This is the challenge of affirmative action in medicine—and this is a challenge our young minority physicians are willing and now able to accept.

SPECIAL PROBLEMS FOR BLACK PHYSICIANS

In 1944, when Gunnar Myrdal wrote "The Negro Problem," he mentioned the particular plight of all Negro business and professional men (322–25). Their exclusion from the larger White market forced them to try to maintain a monopoly over the Negro market. "On the one hand, they find the caste wall blocks their economic and social opportunities. On the other hand, they have, at the same time, a vested interest in racial segregation since it gives them what opportunities they have." Furthermore, "The poverty of the Negro people represents a general limitation of opportunity for Negro businessmen and professionals." These were factors that explained the common observation that Black physicians opposed the development of health clinics in their neighborhoods, despite the obvious need, because these public-health-operated clinics threatened their income. The lack of opportunity to pursue postgraduate training also kept them in a weakened competitive position with White physicians. There were a number of small private Black hospitals in several large urban centers, but in many parts of the South even segregated hospital wings employed only White physicians. In the 1940s Myrdal cited Harlem Hospital Center in New York City as being one of the few examples in the nation where Black and White physicians worked as professional equals in the same hospital.

By 1958 most of these all-Black hospitals were closing down. Black physicians were beginning to get appointments to the medical staffs of White hospitals, and training programs were beginning to open up. These trends have continued. We are now faced with a situation in which not only Black hospitals, but all of the large public hospitals in large urban centers, have already closed or are on the verge of financial collapse.

A case in point is Harlem Hospital Center in New York City, where I was chief of the psychiatry and substance abuse service for almost twenty years. Patients in Harlem do not primarily rely on physicians in private offices; rather they go to hospitals for medical care. In the past they came mainly to Harlem Hospital for general and specialist care. When I arrived in 1982, that hospital had approximately 1,000 beds. In the spring of 2000, the bed capacity was down to 325, and occupancy rates were still problematically low. Even in the psychiatry departments our beds had increased from 53 to 88, but we fell back to 66 beds in May 1998 when our shortened length of stay left us with low occupancy rates. Our residency training program with thirty-four trainees was reduced to seventeen in the year 2000, and the physician attending staff dropped from forty to thirty-five, despite the loss of resident physicians. Other clinical departments suffered an even greater loss of physician and resident staff: Medicine, Surgery, Pediatrics, OB-GYN, and Ambulatory Care. Indices of health care need in central Harlem showed no dramatic improvement: It still had greater health needs than other parts of the city. It also had the greatest number of people, perhaps as many as a third, who had no health care insurance coverage of any kind. Harlem Hospital meantime is operated only on funds it collects primarily through Medicaid (50 percent federal, 25 percent state, and 25 percent city dollars). With the advent of a managed care medical market the future survival of Harlem Hospital and other municipal hospitals is in doubt.

What will this mean in terms of the continued provision of first-rate health care in central Harlem, and first-rate residency training opportunities for Blacks and Hispanic physicians? The answer is clear. The patients already are preferring to go to private voluntary hospitals in neighboring parts of Manhattan. Certainly all patients with any insurance coverage are sought after by New York Presbyterian Hospital, St. Lukes Hospital, and Mt. Sinai Hospital. A small predominantly Black private voluntary hospital in central Harlem, North General Hospital, well staffed by well-trained Black physicians for the most part, is also fighting for fiscal survival.

Who then will train Black residents who have provided a major part of medical care under physician attending supervision? The private voluntary predominantly White hospitals will do so. In my past two decades running a residency training program at Harlem, training close to 250 young physicians, only 6 were African American. Approximately 70 percent were Blacks, but they came from Haiti or other Caribbean countries, or the West African nations. The remaining 30 percent came from India, Pakistan, the Philippines, and several from Russia. It is primarily from these foreign medical school graduates that we recruited many of our physician attending staff as well, although our attending staff has always consisted of as many as one-third who were African American. Blacks graduating from U.S. medical schools for the past two decades have preferred to accept training appointments at the more prestigious teaching hospitals either in New York or other large urban centers.

With this desegregation of medical education and postgraduate training, and medical care, will there be any assurance that these opportunities will remain open? Will Black patients and Black physicians encounter racial prejudice and unfair treatment in these neighboring medical institutions? The future prospects are not so certain as is the actual loss of a predominantly Black medical institutional presence in central Harlem. This brings us to the final chapter, "The Future of Affirmative Action in Medicine." It is my concern that we may be desegregating faster than we are integrating.

VIII. The Future of Affirmative Action

IN MEDICINE

THE PAST THIRTY YEARS have witnessed a remarkable improvement in medical educational opportunity for Black Americans. In this final chapter I outline the nature of these changes, then review the substantial legal and political assault that has been launched against this progress, and summarize the rationale for continuing the effort. Special reference will be made to the implications for Black Americans because the history of our nation, in its early economic beginning, was founded on slave labor. Affirmative action represents a recent attempt to overcome the enduring system of color caste that continues to blight the lives of all Americans. A concluding section deals with the feasibility of success in the recently mounted national affirmative action effort to equalize the health status of African Americans with other ethnic groups.

Table 44 shows that from 1968 to 1997 total medical school enrollment nearly doubled, from just under thirty-six thousand in 1968 to just under sixty-seven thousand in 1997 (AAMC 1978, 299; 1998). Whereas women represented only 8.8 percent of all medical students in 1968, their share increased to 24.3 percent by 1978 and to 42.6 percent in 1997. This spectacular affirmative action achievement for women did not produce a significant political backlash. Indeed the AAMC never officially launched an affirmative action admissions program for women as they did for minority groups in 1970. The program for women was silent, unannounced, but hugely successful. Another little-noted change, similarly unannounced, was among Asian Americans, who went from a little over 2.0 percent of all medical students in 1968 to 18.4 percent by 1997. Among underrepresented minority groups the progress of Black Americans is shown by their growth from 2.2 percent of all medical students in 1968, to 5.7 percent in 1978 and to 7.9 percent in 1997.

This improvement has sparked one of the most impassioned debates in our generation. Black Americans made similar gains in the fields of law, business administration, and engineering, all resulting from race-sensitive admissions programs. It should also be noted that currently more White males are enrolled in medical schools than during pre–affirmative action years, and that all groups benefited from the almost doubling of medical school places from 1968 until now. A rising tide lifted all boats.

In 1980 Blacks represented 11.5 percent of the total United States population of 226 million, but only 3.1 percent of the 433,255 physicians in our nation. A decade later in 1990, Blacks were 11.7 percent of the 249 million total population and now were 3.6 percent of the 586,715 physicians in the United States (AAMC 1998). Blacks are still far from being represented equally among our nation's physicians. Projections of the nation's physician workforce suggest that it may be another fifty years before the proportion of Black physicians achieves parity with the proportion in the general population (Watson 1999).

In 1968 Howard and Meharry enrolled approximately 85 percent of all Black American medical students. By 1997, two new predominantly Black medical schools had been established: Morehouse School of Medicine in Atlanta, which was founded in 1978, and the Charles R. Drew University of Medicine and Science, which admitted its first class in 1981. The total number of Black Americans enrolled in these four schools in 1998 was 712, or 13.4 percent of all Black American medical students, distributed as follows: Howard 125, Meharry 301, Morehouse 123, and Drew 23 (AAMC 1998). This represents a dramatic desegregation of medical education over the past thirty years.

TABLE 44.　Total Enrollment in U.S. Medical Schools, 1968, 1978, 1997

	1968		1978		1997	
	Total	%	Total	%	Total	%
Number of Schools	99		124		127	
Total Students	35,833		62,242		66,900	
Men	32,697		47,149		38,395	57.4
Women	3,136	8.8	15,113	24.3	28,505	42.6
Underrepresented minorities	854	2.4	4,901	7.9	8,178	12.2
Black	783	2.2	3,540	5.7	5,303	7.9
Mexican American	59	0.2	882	1.4	1,838	2.8
Native American	9	0.03	202	0.3	561	0.8
Puerto Rican (Mainland)	3	.008	277	0.5	476	0.7
All others	932	2.6	3,595	5.8	14,828[a]	22.2

Source: AAMC enrollment data for 1968, 1978, 1997.

[a]Asian or Pacific Islander = 12,303, or 83%, of total.

AFFIRMATIVE ACTION IN MEDICAL EDUCATION

A number of specific anti–affirmative action lawsuits and new laws have created heated controversy (Bergeison and Cantor 1999).

1. In 1995 the University of California regents decided to prohibit the use of race, religion, sex, color, ethnicity, or national origin as a criterion for admission effective January 1, 1997.
2. Proposition 209 in California and Initiative 200 in the State of Washington were passed by voters respectively in 1996 and 1998 prohibiting race-sensitive admissions, public employment, or public contracting.
3. *Hopwood v. Texas* in 1997 forbade the University of Texas from using race as an admission criterion, a decision by the Fifth Circuit Court of Appeals, which covers also Mississippi and Louisiana.
4. In December 1998 the First Circuit Court of Appeals, in *Wessman v. Gittens,* ruled that an admissions set-aside for minority applicants at Boston Latin School was unconstitutional (this action brought these suits to the secondary school level).
5. Two pending class action cases against the University of Michigan, *Grantz et al. v. Bollinger* and *Grutter v. Bollinger,* challenged the use of race in admissions decisions in the undergraduate and law schools.

Some of these, and other expected legal challenges, are aimed not only at state-operated colleges and universities, but also at private institutions that receive federal funds of any kind. Programs for minority high school students only that help them to become better prepared for college would also be curtailed. Indeed some of these opponents would be against any kind of special program to enhance the acceptance chances of minority students, viewing them as reverse discrimination against Whites. Blacks would thereby be locked permanently into an underclass status.

In the May 7, 2001, issue of the *American Prospect,* Alexander Wohl calls these reverses to affirmative action "Diversity on Trial." He called attention to litigation against the University of Michigan's admission policy. On December 13, 2000, a federal district judge appointed by Ronald Reagan upheld the constitutionality of race-conscious undergraduate admissions to the Michigan undergraduate school. Three months later in the same district court another Reagan appointee, Judge Bernard Friedman, held that the race-conscious admission program at the university's law school was unconstitutional. Some observers particularly stressed the seriousness of Judge Friedman's opinion that it has not been shown that there is a compelling state interest in assuring ethnic diversity in a class, that "race-neutral" alternatives to affirmative action should have been tried, including "decreasing the emphasis for all applicants on undergraduate GPA and LSAT scores, using a lottery system for all qualified applicants, or a system whereby a certain percentage of the top graduates from various colleges or universities are admitted." This abandonment of objective standards of academic measurement is precisely what has occurred in California, Florida, and Texas in the wake of attacks on race-sensitive affirmative action. Since the quality of schools varies so widely, the top schools in the state systems could find themselves admitting less qualified students and minority students might choose to attend less competitive segregated schools to increase their chances of admission, in short, lowering academic standards in the premier state university units (Selengo 2001; Rosen 2001).

This adverse Michigan decision, combined with the adverse decision in 1996 ruling against the University of Texas law school admissions for minority applicants and the favorable decision on the University of Washington's law school admissions in 2000, made it appear increasingly likely that this issue will be brought to the Supreme Court soon. Matters became still more clouded on May 14, 2002, when the U.S. Court of Appeals for the Sixth Circuit said it was not yet ready to rule on the lawsuit involving undergraduate admissions but decided 5 to 4 to overturn a lower court's ruling that the University of Michigan's law school had illegally discriminated against White applicants. The court said the university had considered race appropriately in trying to enroll a "critical mass" of minority students to contribute to educational diversity (Schmidt 2002).

The basic legal ambiguity is derived from the Supreme Court's decision in 1978 in the case of *Regents of the University of California v. Bakke*. Justices Brennan, White, Marshall, and Blackmun would have supported the use of a quota to give equal opportunity under the Fourteenth Amendment, while another four justices opposed race-conscious admissions under federal law—Justices Stevens, Stewart, Rehnquist, and Chief Justice Warren Burger. Justice Lewis Powell's majority opinion was that while quotas setting aside admission places were not permissible, race can be considered as one factor in making admissions decisions in order to promote diversity and an improved educational experience for all students in a class. Because "diversity" and "Academic freedom," a First Amendment concern, were the basis for Powell's decision and none of the other justices took that precise stand, there is confusion concerning how the present Supreme Court would decide.

Wohl (2001) and others are fairly certain that Chief Justice Rehnquist will be joined by Justices Scalia and Thomas, who are believed to be strongly opposed to affirmative action, and possibly Kennedy, who has "shown great skepticism about affirmative action in previous cases." On the other side, Justices Ginsburg, Breyer, and Souter would likely be joined by Stevens, who has not concluded that race can "ever be used as a factor in an admissions decision." For these reasons it is speculated that Justice Sandra O'Connor might make the decision on the constitutionality of minority admissions. Her previous decisions opposing affirmative action set-asides in business contracts and employment were, in her own words, not to be taken as opposition to "achieving diversity in public graduate schools." Justice O'Connor is believed to favor the stand of former justice Powell in preferring to favor a decision based on a limited scope such as "diversity" rather than the broader scope of the Fourteenth Amendment's equal protection clause.

Reminding us that the Supreme Court's *Brown v. Board of Education* in 1954 found segregated schools unconstitutional, with all justices concurring that they violated the fourteenth Amendment's equal protection clause, and that the following year Brown II recommended that desegregation proceed with "all deliberate speed," James Patterson in his recent book concludes that within ten years most southern schools had become nominally desegregated. Its effects were nullified by southern Whites flight to the suburbs, setting up private schools and setting up ability-tracking systems that kept the races apart even within the same school. Segregation still prevailed in the North through de facto residential segregation. For all these reasons the academic achievement gap between Black and White child persists, and little is being done nationally to fight continued racially segregated neighborhoods (J. T. Patterson 2000). We should bear this in mind as we speculate on the possible consequences of how the present Supreme Court may rule on cases soon to come before it on affirmative action in higher education. Whether the court decides positively or negatively will not necessarily matter very much. The Warren Court realized in the 1950s that "courts by themselves could not greatly change American society."

PROBLEMS IN PREPARING MINORITY STUDENTS FOR ADMISSION

Since it began operations in 1972 the Robert Wood Johnson Foundation has supported programs to increase the enrollment of minority medical students as well as the development of minority faculty. Specifically, the Minority Medical Education Program (MMEP) provides an intensive six-week residential summer program for minority premedical students to enhance the likelihood of their being accepted. At eight different medical schools these students receive training to improve their science course preparation, hone test-taking and communication skills, and learn the fine points of the application process. As of 1991 nearly half of all U.S. medical schools sponsored some variety of preprofessional programs. Minority students applying for acceptance into the MMEP are required to complete a process that closely parallels the one they will complete later, through the American Medical College Application Service (AMCAS), which provides uniform application forms and procedures and is used by almost all medical schools.

Applicants to MMEP must submit their undergraduate college admission test scores, transcripts of grades, a personal statement of their interest in a medical career, and letters of recommendation. A minimum grade point average of 3.0 (on a 4.0 scale) is expected, including at least a 2.75 in the science courses and a score of at least 950 on the Scholastic Aptitude Test (SAT). Since applicants are expected to show these threshold levels of academic potential, the program does not actually increase the pipeline of acceptable minority applicants. A short-term six-week program could not develop an unprepared student. In collaboration with the Association of American Medical Colleges (AAMC), the Prematriculation questionnaire, which provides information on the applicant's family background, is administered along with the Medical College Admission Test (MCAT). Minority students participating in the foundation-sponsored preparatory program could be compared with minority premedical students who had not participated. Between the summers of 1989 and 1997 the Robert Wood Johnson MMEP had served 6,479 students, of whom 48.7 percent applied to medical schools, and 63 percent of those applicants were accepted. Acceptance rates for MMEP students were higher even after controlling for college grades and MCAT scores, and were as great for those who participated after their freshman or sophomore year as the upper division years. The six-week program also was demonstrably more effective with minority students who had relatively higher grades or MCAT scores. These favorable effects were maintained even in 1996 and 1997 after affirmative action litigation created a less welcoming environment (Bergeison and Cantor 1999; Cantor, Bergeison, and Baker 1998).

In 1991 the AAMC launched its program to admit three thousand underrepresented minorities (URM) by the year 2000. The target was 19 percent of all new medical school matriculants, equal to the proportion of underrepresented minorities in the U.S. population. Medical schools were encouraged to form linkages with minority high school students interested in a medical career and performing well academically, and also with colleges graduating large numbers of minority premed students. However, from 1994 with 2,014 first-year students, there was a drop in 1995 to 2,010 (Division of Community and Minority Programs 1996). The number continued to decline, to 1,770 in 1997, the lowest since 1991. After reaching a second high in 1994, URM new entrants declined from 12.4 percent to 10.9 percent of all entering medical students. This drop was specifically related to adverse affirmative action: Proposition 209 caused a 16 percent decline in California schools, a 29 percent decline in Texas, and a 13 percent decline in Mississippi and Louisiana, all states adversely affected by the *Hopwood* decision (AAMC 1998, 8–9).

Table 45 illustrates the downward trend of URM admissions during the past decade, 1990 through 1999. Unless new programs are mounted, we can anticipate further stagnation or decline in the decade to come. Not shown in this table is the fact that Black women are increasing their numbers, while Black men are progressively declining. As Theodore Cross and Robert Slater have shown (2000), up until the mid-1970s Black men earned nearly 75 percent of all professional degrees awarded to African Americans, but Black men won only 47 percent of all professional degrees in 1991 and 42 percent in 1997; Black men in 1977 won 60 percent of all doctorates but only 35 percent in 1998.

Specifically in medicine, in the decade of the 1990s, in 1994 of 1,384 Blacks admitted, only 550, or about 40 percent, were men, but in 1999 only 406 of the 1,199, or 34 percent, were men. While women of all groups are increasing their share of medical school admissions, their proportion still does not match that of men: in 1999 men were 54 percent of the 117 Native Americans admitted, 54 percent of 415 Mexican Americans, 50 percent of the 119 Mainland Puerto Ricans. Among Whites, of 11,030 admitted, 57 percent were men, in what continues to be a profession dominated by men.

TABLE 45. First-Year Underrepresented Minority Entrants to U.S. Medical Schools, 1990–99

	1990	1991	1992	1993	1994	1995	1996	1997	1998	1999
Black	1,104	1,147	1,262	1,350	1,384	1,365	1,266	1,202	1,269	1,119
Native American	72	102	121	138	134	152	154	137	155	117
Mexican American	281	328	427	399	476	504	470	418	435	415
Puerto Rican (Mainland)	105	125	118	105	136	116	146	116	111	119
Total	1,562	1,702	1,928	1,992	2,130	2,137	2,036	1,873	1,970	1,770

As Cross and Slater emphasize, the decline in the proportion of men in higher education in general took hold much earlier for Blacks than for Whites. One reason for this decline may be the possibility that recruiting Black women improves affirmative action targets both for gender and ethnicity. More basic causes may be the erosion of the Black family; in more than two-thirds of all Black households there is no father or other strong role model. The culture of the primary and secondary school system appears to favor young Black girls over boys since teachers, predominantly female, see more Black boys who are disciplinary problems. An antiachievement ethic may therefore have become more prevalent among male Blacks. Media portrayal of successful Black men concentrates on athletes and entertainers, occupations requiring little formal education, sending "large numbers of young Black males down a career-blind alley," to quote Cross and Slater. Educational enrichment programs aimed to attract larger proportions of Black males must therefore overcome special cultural hurdles.

Several medical schools have assumed the responsibility of increasing the pool of qualified minority applicants. The most noteworthy of them, perhaps, is the Gateway to Higher Education sponsored by the City University of New York Medical School (Slater and Iler 1991). This is a comprehensive four-year high school program with specially designed enrichments and supports. Established in 1986, the program is demonstrating that minority students in the ninth grade who are performing at least at grade level can show outstanding scholastic achievement by the time of high school graduation.

In 1990, the first 119 graduates of this program were freshmen at sixty different colleges and universities nationwide: two-thirds of the Gateway graduates scored 500 or better in the SAT mathematics section, 25 percent scored over 600, and all of them exceeded the national average on the SAT verbal section. The students responded positively to the increased demands, attendance at classes was nearly perfect, and only three dropped out of high school. The program, developed by Dr. Alfred Gellhorn while he was dean of the medical school, is a collaborative venture with the New York City Board of Education and is funded by a special state grant and private foundations at an average annual cost of twelve hundred dollars per student beyond the basic educational allotment.

Total enrollment in 1990 was six hundred students from five high schools. A junior high school component was added in 1990, so that more than one thousand students were participating in Gateway. The value of the program is illustrated by one finding: for Black students taking the SAT in that first graduating year, those in the Gateway had a mean total score of

978.3, while Black students nationally scored 737. However, if one wanted to be skeptical, one might suggest the Gateway students are more highly motivated and from more highly motivated families than average and therefore the program is just skimming off the better students who would have performed above average anyway. The medical school employs two full-time directors who collaborate with fifteen teachers at each participating school who are selected for their special interest in the program's goals. Three additional university-based professional level staff assist part time in scheduling special laboratory, computer tutorials, guidance, and development of a parent council interchange with teachers.

A ten-year follow-up by Iler and Slater (1998) showed continuing success of this program in sending high proportions of these students into college and professional careers in medicine, sciences, engineering, and technology. Their goal is to have 15 percent of their graduates entering medical school, and they have achieved 7 percent, approximately one-half of this goal, with their first graduates. In a national AAMC survey of minority students at high school level interested in pursuing a medical career, 47 percent of all of the New York state students were in the Gateway program (Iler and Slater 1998).

The Gateway program does not come close to the spectacular success of Xavier University, the only Black college affiliated with the Roman Catholic Church. The Xavier program is not under medical school auspices. Xavier was founded in 1915 in New Orleans by Katherine Drexel and the Sisters of the Blessed Sacrament at the request of the local archbishop, specifically because of the limited higher educational opportunity for Black youth (*Handbook of Historically Black Colleges and Universities* 1999, 109). With a current enrollment of 850 men and 1,973 women, Xavier for a number of years has been number one nationally in placing Black students in medical schools. In the year 2000 the top ten schools in producing Black first-year enrollees were Xavier (73); Morehouse (31); Howard University (26); Spelman (24); Johns Hopkins (19); Harvard (17); Hampton University (16); Oakwood College in Huntsville, Alabama, which is affiliated with the Seventh Day Adventist Church (16); University of Maryland–College Park (16); University of California–Los Angeles (15). Major reasons for Xavier's success are the more than thirty years of continuous administrative leadership provided by its premedical student adviser, Dr. J. W. Carmichael, and Dr. Norman Francis, president of the university, and the more than $84 million and public and private grants received in just the five-year period from 1995–2000. Not only has Xavier sought out high school students interested in a career in medicine or other sciences, but the college has provided programs to improve the quality of teachers of those subjects in New Orleans high schools. On entering Xavier all premed students take a prescribed core curriculum not only in science but also in nonscience subjects, a curriculum that is taught to meet national standards, all of which requires unprecedented cooperation from the faculty. In addition to the seventy-three Xavier students who went to medical school another eighty-seven went on to pursue graduate degree work in science-related fields (Stewart 2000, 22–26).

Significant programs for scholastic development such as Gateway and at Xavier University are crucial for the future success of affirmative action and other scientific fields because increasing the pool of students in the pipeline is the key. States and localities that have been responsible for providing inferior education for children in minority communities in the past should accept a legal and moral responsibility to do the right thing.

In 1996 the Association of American Medical Colleges leadership issued an important policy statement reaffirming their commitment to affirmative action recruitment programs as essential to desegregate and diversify our national physician manpower, and for the purposes of improving not only the education of all students, but also the quality of health care and medical research affecting all segments of our society (Nickens and Cohen 1996). Nathan Glazer (1999), in a reversal from his previous position, now maintains that for African Americans, racial group membership alone produces handicaps that result in lower test scores that understate their academic potential, which would be revealed if they gained access to superior education. U.S. academic leadership, he contends, is overwhelmingly committed to continue these programs, as they offer the best hope that our nation will ever become a color-blind society of equals.

MEASURING MERIT

Considerable misunderstanding exists about what test scores and grade point averages mean in the evaluation of medical school applicants in a given year. Let us look more closely at what happens.

In 1997 there were 43,020 applicants for 16,165 places in the entering classes of all of the 127 medical schools (AAMC 1998). This means that the chance of being accepted overall was 38 percent. What we are not told is how many of these applicants were well enough qualified to have been accepted. We must realize that almost every one of the 43,000 applicants believes he or she is qualified. Each of them has graduated from college with grade point averages and test scores that seemed to them, and perhaps to their premed faculty adviser, to be adequate. In fact the premed adviser will usually have advised the student to apply to three different kinds of schools, probably four to which the student has a chance of being accepted, four to which the student almost certainly will be accepted, and four to which the student has only a slim chance of being admitted. Premed advisers have usually had some years of experience in discerning the behavior of different schools, and premed students have family members or friends who are eager to share their knowledge and conjectures about an applicant's chances at a given school.

Let us try to put ourselves in the position of members of an admissions committee. Recall again that while one out of three applicants is admitted, most often at least two of the three applicants could have been acceptable based on grade point average and scores and even interview and other subjective judgments of their potential. Admissions committees face a much more daunting challenge when it comes to the more highly selective and high-prestige medical schools. Even for schools not in the highest prestige category, the problem of selecting students is great indeed. For example in 1997 Boston University had 10,632 applicants for the 151 places in its freshman class, meaning that an applicant had on average a 1.4 percent chance of being accepted. Harvard had 3,708 applicants for 165 places (a 4.4 percent chance). Does this mean then the average applicant has a better chance of being accepted at Harvard than at BU? Not at all. Rather, it means that more students felt they had a chance for admission to BU than to Harvard and that Harvard's applicants had probably been more carefully self-selected and carefully advised. It would not be remarkable to find that as many as 98 percent of Harvard's and probably 85 percent of BU's applicants are qualified, based not only on grades and test scores but subjective evaluations of the applicant's future potential as a physician. The admissions committees at both Boston University and Harvard reject thousands of well-qualified applicants every year, and they must have a rationale for these decisions.

In 1997 Boston University received applications from 368 Black Americans, 140 men and 328 women; 19 were accepted, of whom 7 were men and 12 women. Of that group, 9 matriculated, 3 men and 6 women. Their first-year class was therefore 6 percent Black, but this could only have reflected an institutional commitment to have a Black presence in their entering class of 151. Almost certainly only a fraction of these students would have been admitted on the basis of test scores and grades alone and fewer still using a lottery system, quite aside from the fact that at both schools many qualified minority and nonminority students were not admitted. That same year Harvard had 216 Black applicants; 27 were accepted, of whom 12 were men and 15 women. Of those 27 who were accepted, 15 chose to come to Harvard, 7 men and 8 women. Harvard's entering class of 165 therefore was 9.1 percent Black. My reading of this occurrence was that Harvard was expressing a continued leadership commitment to admit and graduate a significant number of Black physicians.

As future physicians, the majority of students will be practitioners. Some will be teachers, a few others will be researchers, while still others will be administrators, but almost all will combine several of these areas. Test scores and grades alone cannot substitute for more comprehensive indices, based on past life performance and interview behavior, of the kind of physician this candidate could become if given an opportunity to be a member of that class for four years.

Choosing the members of a new medical school class is a serious undertaking that carries long-standing social consequences. Society gives the medical profession what amounts almost to a monopoly right to care for those who are sick and injured or dying, and the right to inquire about the most personal and private details of a patient's life in the interest of assessing and treating their health problems. In carrying out their mission of health care, physicians are expected to be able to form rapid, helpful, personal communicating relationships with patients and members of their families. Physicians also are expected to be able to work collaboratively with other members of the health care team, nurses, social workers, lawyers, members of the news media, clergy, and other community leaders. All this and more is to be done with competence, compassion, integrity, humility and in a manner that instills hope and trust in others.

In making selections of the students who will make up the class, a conscious effort should be made to include members who represent all components of the community. Let us say that you are on the faculty of a medical school; you would certainly be concerned that no student be admitted who is not competent to handle the academic demands of the curriculum; otherwise the student will not graduate. If a student has gone to a first-rate college and graduated with a B average, has a medical college admission test score high enough to predict a 95 percent or higher chance of graduating, looks good in interviews, and has a life history of overcoming obstacles or of showing signs of resourcefulness, creativity, or leadership potential, the student is a good candidate for admission. The problem is that you have an embarrassment of riches. Perhaps as many as 80 percent or more of White applicants and Asian candidates meet those criteria. At least 40 percent to 50 percent of Black applicants have the same qualifications. However, since you have only 100 places in the entering class, but several thousand qualified applicants, you must reject many qualified applicants. You will want to have a class that reflects equal and fair treatment of men and women, persons of differing religious and ethnic backgrounds, and social class and regional origins. You will be guided by considerations of the value of diversity within the class whose members will be with each other for four years and who in the future will be providing a crucial human service to all members of the public for the next fifty years or more.

In years past, most of the leading medical schools had an informal quota, admitting only an occasional Black student. The University of Michigan, from which I graduated as the only Black student in the class of 1946, had graduated one or two or three Black students almost every year since 1872, making it one of the schools with an enlightened admissions policy. Except for Howard and Meharry, the quota for Blacks in most schools nationwide was less than 1 percent. When I joined the Cornell faculty in 1968, I learned that from its beginning in 1898, Cornell had graduated only twelve blacks, six of whom had come from Africa rather than the United States. I also learned from discussions with physicians who had attended Cornell in earlier years that until the 1940s, Cornell had an unofficial quota of only about 5 percent Jews and 10 percent Catholics in its first-year class. Each incoming class also contained between 5 percent and 10 percent women. Similar admission patterns were practiced in almost all of the nation's medical schools.

All of this changed gradually and then changed more rapidly following World War II. Jewish applicants no longer are held to a low quota and now comprise large, and unpublicized, portions of all medical school classes. The same schools also opened up silently to Catholics. These gender- and religious-based restrictions had nothing to do with merit or demerit, but simply reflected general American institutional prejudice and bigotry in earlier years. Medical schools never admitted that they had a quota for limiting the numbers of Jews, Catholics, or women, although by law Blacks were excluded from southern and some border states' schools. We have observed the opening up of medical schools for women who went from 8.7 percent of first-year students in 1968 to 42.6 percent in 1997, again a favorable change that will bring untold benefits to our entire nation. All of these demographic and more democratic changes in the nation's medical workforce are now perceived as fair. The Women's Medical College of Pennsylvania became coeducational and changed its name to the Medical College of Pennsylvania when its mission began to be carried out in all medical schools.

Ludmerer explains that the low percentage of women in medicine, which for decades had been stable at between 6 and 7 percent, compared favorably with the low percentages in such fields as law or engineering, both at the 2 percent level. In the late 1960s women began to enter most of these professions from which they had been informally excluded, primarily as a result of the women's movement for civil rights, as well as legal protection of these rights by enactment of the 1972 Title IX of the Higher Education Amendments banning sex discrimination in education programs receiving federal funds. Once women were admitted their medical school presence did not plateau in the mid-1970s, as it did for minority students, because the educational pipeline for women was as strong as it was for men and the vast majority of women admitted also were White (Ludmerer 1999, 256–57).

A profile of all the entering class of 1996 reveals that 34.5 percent of the 46,968 applicants to medical school were accepted. On average they made about a dozen applications, and they received almost two acceptances each, although this varies by subgroup to which they belong. The acceptance rate for Blacks was 34.7 percent, for Whites 37.8 percent, for women 34.5 percent, for Asians 32.6 percent. The grade point average for the groups mentioned above were Blacks 3.1 in science subjects and 3.4 in all other subjects; for Whites, the science grade point average was 3.5 and 3.6 for all other subjects; for Asians 3.6 for science subjects and 3.7 for other subjects. You can be certain that some students with grade point averages of 3.9 or even 4.0 were rejected because they were less promising candidates for other reasons. Wide differences were found in the Medical College Admission Test scores: verbal reasoning for Blacks, 7.8 on a scale up to 15, for Whites, 9.9, for Asians, 9.6; physical sciences: Blacks, 7.6, Whites, 10.1, Asians, 10.7; biological sciences: Black, 7.9, White, 10.2, Asian, 10.7 (AAMC 1998).

The experience of most medical schools reveals that a score of 7.0 on a fifteen-point scale is high enough to predict a 95 percent or higher graduation rate, especially if the student has graduated from a first-rate college with a grade point average of B or better. Scores of 13, 14, or 15 do not forecast graduate rates any better. Prior to 1977 an older medical college admission test had been used for twenty-six years. Scores on that test ranged up to 800. The four subscales for the old MCAT were Verbal, Quantitative, General Information, and Science. The proportion of students dismissed or repeating the first year is given in 50-point ranges of subscale scores. For those in the 450–99 range, the failure rate ranged from 8 percent (Quantitative) to a low of 4 percent (Verbal). The 500–49 range went from a high of 5 percent (Quantitative) to 3 percent (Verbal and General Information).

The 550–99 range went from a high of 3 percent (in Verbal, Quantitative, and General Information) to a low of 2 percent (Science). In the 600–49 range, the high of 3 percent (Quantitative) was seen with a low of 2 percent in Verbal, General Information, and Science. For the higher ranges 650–99 and 700–99 the same 2 percent failure rate was uniformly found on all four subscales. Essentially those scoring in the 550–99 range had no more than a 2 percent to 3 percent failure rate, which was similar to that of those scoring higher, up to 799. Admissions committees in various geographic areas were, in consultation with other faculty, free to decide the risk level they could tolerate, given the strength of their total applicant pool. (Data on MCAT scores are from Appendix G-7 in Carnegie Council 1977 [237], which is based on AAMC data.) Careful studies showed that students scoring 450 to 500 had graduation rates of 97 percent to 98 percent, and that those who scored 600 to 800 did not have higher success. In other words, beyond a certain criterion score, the numbers have no significant predictive power in graduation rates. A few students will drop out for reasons having nothing to do with cognitive ability as measured by admissions test scores. In my opinion, the scores do predict which students have had the benefit of high-quality schooling and competition with other bright students. Parental characteristics by race were as follows: Occupation: professional or managerial category for fathers of Blacks, was 51.5 percent, Whites in that category 61.4 percent, Asian 60.1 percent. Father having a college degree: Blacks, 14.1 percent, Whites, 18.7 percent, Asian, 16.6 percent. Mother having a college degree: Blacks, 15.0 percent, Whites, 24.1 percent, Asians, 31.7 percent. Median parental income: Blacks, $50,000, Whites, $75,000, Asians, $70,000. Fathers who were physicians: Blacks, 1.5 percent, Whites, 1.8 percent, Asians, 10.1 percent.

Despite obviously different life circumstances of Blacks, lower grade point averages and even relatively lower MCAT scores provide the basis for legal challenge to their being admitted fairly. This is the crux of the argument against race-sensitive admissions.

AFFIRMATIVE ACTION IN AMERICAN HIGHER EDUCATION

The Affirmative Action admission of Black Americans to the nation's medical schools has been a part of the larger movement to consider race as one of the factors favoring admission of qualified candidates to colleges and universities from which they were largely excluded for the past four hundred years. Americans are deeply divided over this issue, and until recently the debate has been little guided by hard evidence. In 1998, therefore, the issue was greatly clarified by the publication of the long-term consequences of considering race in college and university admissions. William Bowen, president of the Mellon Foundation and former president of Princeton University, and Derek Bok, former president of Harvard University and former dean of the Harvard Law School, drew on a huge database containing the admissions and transcript records and subsequent occupational histories of more than eighty thousand undergraduate students who matriculated at twenty-eight selective colleges and universities from 1951 to 1989 (Bowen and Bok 1998). The aim of the study was to obtain a long-term view of differences between Black and White students from high school through undergraduate, graduate, and professional school, and into their occupational and community life. The authors picked the most selective research universities and liberal arts colleges because they are the schools that have been attacked for presumably admitting less qualified Blacks while rejecting more highly qualified Whites. The Bowen-Bok calculations showed that if admissions had been based entirely on grades and test scores, Black enrollment at these colleges would drop by 50 to 70 percent and from 7 percent to 2 percent of total enrollment (51).

Critics had surmised that Black students would become demoralized finding themselves competing with White students who had higher grades and scores, and that the Black students would be more successful in less competitive colleges. However, Bowen and Bok found that these Black students with the lowest SAT scores had higher graduation rates than Blacks who attended less competitive colleges. A striking finding was that the average SAT scores of Black entrants to the most selective schools in 1989 were higher than the average of all matriculants in the same institutions in 1951, an observation that middle-aged and elderly alumni of those colleges should note. In other words, test scores of Whites have steadily increased from one generation to the next (30).

Despite differences in test scores on admission, both Blacks and Whites highly valued their experience studying and living together during their college years. How well the Black students performed after college also was very impressive. Forty percent went on to earn graduate or professional school degrees, compared with 37 percent of White students who entered the 28 colleges in 1976. From all colleges nationally, only 8 percent of Blacks and 12 percent of Whites go on to attain doctoral or professional degrees. A further breakdown of the Bowen-Bok graduates from the group of elite schools showed that for the 1976 entering cohort, 14 percent of Blacks and 11 percent of Whites received law degrees, 11 percent of Blacks and 8 percent of Whites received medical degrees, 13 percent of Blacks and

13 percent of Whites got business degrees, and 4 percent of Blacks and 7 percent of Whites were awarded Ph.D. degrees (100). Bowen and Bok constructed a profile of 700 Black students who matriculated in 1976 but who would have been rejected under a color-blind standard (281). More than 225 went on to attain professional degrees or doctorates, about 70 are now physicians and 60 are lawyers, 125 are business executives, more than 300 are leaders in civic activities. The average earnings of the group exceed $71,000, which, according to census data, is at least 75 percent more than Blacks who hold bachelor's degrees in their age cohort but not as high as their White former classmates. Two-thirds of this group considered themselves "very satisfied" with their undergraduate years. However, the Black students tended to earn slightly lower grades than Whites with the same SAT scores.

Some have suggested that if these same highly selective colleges had admitted students from low-income families by preference, without regard to race, the same result would be achieved and with less adverse public opinion. Bowen and Bok disagree. Although 50 percent of American Black families with children sixteen to eighteen years old fall into the lowest of three socioeconomic categories (neither parent has a college degree and family income is below $22,000), only 14 percent of Black students in their study were from such families. While only 3 percent of all Black families are in the highest category (defined as at least one parent being a college graduate and family income is more than $70,000), 15 percent of Black students in this study were from such families. The authors point out that in absolute numbers there would be six times as many Whites as Black students in the low-income pool (51). Further, students from extremely impoverished family backgrounds of any race are usually unable to survive in a highly competitive college environment.

Still others maintain that race-sensitive admissions violate the rights of innocent Whites who are rejected despite their better credentials as shown by grades and test scores. Such injury is small indeed, as Bowen and Bok estimate, inasmuch as if no Blacks were admitted to any of the 28 elite colleges in the study, the chances of admission for any individual White applicant would at most increase from 25 percent to 26.5 percent because there are so many rejected White candidates with the same grades and test scores. On the other hand, the mission of our great universities is not to preserve and solidify the continued exclusion of Black Americans from positions of power and leadership. As Ronald Dworkin pointed out in his review of Bowen and Bok's book (1998), our schools "have traditionally aimed to help improve the collective life of the community, not just by protecting and enhancing its culture and science, or improving its medicine, commerce and agriculture, but by helping to make that collective life more just and harmonious . . . the continuity and debilitating segregation of the United States by race, class, occupation and status is an enemy of both justice and harmony. . . . Affirmative action has begun to invade that segregation in ways no other program or policy probably could" (100–102).

THE NEED FOR AFFIRMATIVE ACTION AT ELEMENTARY AND HIGH SCHOOL LEVELS

African American children start their education with significant socioeconomic disadvantages compared with European American children: twice as many are low-birthweight babies (10.4 percent v 5.1 percent); nearly 44 percent live in households with annual incomes of less than ten thousand dollars, compared with 9.5 percent European Americans; 66 percent live in single-parent homes, compared with 15.8 percent European Americans; and fewer African American parents have four or more years of high school (68.7 versus 77.6 percent) (*New York Public Library* 1999, 203). Tests of developmental abilities of preschool children show that African Americans score equally well on motor and social and memory scales but score slightly less well on verbal scales. However, African American children begin to lag behind during grade school, and the learning achievement gap remains constant or widens from then on.

The successful outcome in the Supreme Court case of *Brown v. Board of Education* in 1954 put an end to legalized segregated public education. The court ruled that racially segregated schools, legalized in the 1896 Supreme Court *Plessy v. Ferguson* case, had to be ended because they violated the equal protection rights of Black children, who were entitled to receive an equal quality of education that was not possible under conditions of forced segregation. Unfortunately, the years since 1954 have witnessed more segregated school experiences for Black children. Residential segregation has increased since the 1950s, carrying with it not only segregated neighborhoods both in cities and suburbs, but also de facto racially segregated schools (Orfield and Eaton 1996, 53–72; Meier, Stewart, and Eagland 1989, 136–49).

These developments have led many African American leaders to question the wisdom of continuing to seek integration from White Americans who do not want to live with them as neighbors or to have their children attend their schools (Steinberg 1989, 253–302; O. Patterson 1997, 171–203; Allen and Jewell 1995).

While I think it is too early to give up on the goal of achieving racially integrated neighborhoods, it seems obvious that we must either make headway toward that aim or expect an increasingly angry and violent demand for a genuinely separate and equal African American nation within a nation (Canty 1969, 59–73; Klinker and Smith 1999, 317–51).

Amid all this noisy rancor and polarized rhetoric, we may not be addressing the main problem facing us as a single nation. While many Whites feel secure that their children are receiving an education that is relatively superior to what is offered to Blacks, we have serious deficits in the quality of education received by all American children. The problem is spelled in graphic detail in an important book *The State of Americans* (Ceci 1996). Both thirteen-year-olds and seventeen-year-olds scored slightly higher on mathematics and reading tests in 1990 than in 1971 performance, but nearly all of the upward gain of the past twenty years has been due to the extremely large gains made by Black thirteen- and seventeen-year-olds. Changes in the test scores of White students over this same period have been minimal. In 1971 Black students averaged 35 to 40 percentage points below White students; by 1990 the gap has been reduced to 17 to 25 points. Ceci believes that the gains for Black children may be due to the improving educational achievement of Black parents, who now graduate from high school at almost the same rate as Whites, the fact that increasing numbers of Blacks are attending desegregated colleges, and that the average size of nonwelfare families has dropped dramatically in the past twenty years.

Most disturbing are his data on international comparisons of American student test scores in mathematics and science. American fourth graders have gone from the middle of a group of seventeen developed countries to near the bottom. They ranked fourth in 1970 but had dropped to twelfth by the mid-1980s. The picture for American eighth graders is even worse: they were near the bottom in 1970 (fifteenth out of seventeen) and have remained there in the mid-1980s. American schools report only 15 percent of high school seniors taking calculus, although more than half of high school seniors in England and Wales, Israel, Scotland, and Japan take this course. U.S. calculus scores are lowest on international tests: the average score is "less than half that of the children of its major trading partners" (Ceci 1996, 198). In international comparisons our best students do poorly: "the top 10% and top 25% of American students tend to be nearer the achievement levels of Italy and Thailand than to Japan, Sweden and England" (200). Ceci speculates that one main reason for their performance is American children spend much less time in learning activity inside and outside the classroom: for example 21 percent of our nine-year-olds spend more than five hours per weekday watching television, "far more than the children of U.S. trading partners" (201).

Diane Ravitch (1995, 177–86) gives an authoritative presentation of the issues surrounding our failure to develop a national commitment to provide all American children a high-quality education that will make us competitive with the rest of the developed world. First and foremost, most parents are satisfied with the education their children receive, even though increasingly it has become a high-priority political item. Problems arise because the federal government supplies only about 7 percent of the money spent to educate our children, with the rest provided by localities and states that insist on local control of school policy. Because there is fear and mistrust of federal government control of education policy, Congress fails to arrive at bipartisan programs to improve the educational performance of our schools. There is no political consensus that we should have a national standard curriculum and require all children in all parts of the country to be able to pass uniform proficiency tests. Until this is done, there is little likelihood that equal educational opportunity will become a fact in American life. Only then, however, will we be able to demonstrate that we can educate our children as well as other developed nations currently are doing. We have a firm belief that only a fraction of our children are bright by innate good fortune, and that only these children should be placed on a special track and provided a high level of schooling. Ravitch and others point out that this is not a commonly accepted view in many industrialized countries, which assume that all children should be challenged to learn even difficult subjects. Only following this more inclusive principle will it be possible to maximize the more complete potential of a greater proportion of children. Ravitch also points out that by and large, American parents and children are satisfied with the amount of time and hard work their children spend on the academic mission of schools. Our future ability to compete with the next generation of this global village, in this new information age, will be determined largely by our making a national commitment to educational excellence and equality.

THE FUTURE OF COLOR CASTE

The gaps between Black and White test scores, family income (and the much larger gap in wealth), health and longevity are all reflections of the enduring system of color caste, almost 100 years after Black people were freed from slavery, which had lasted 250 years. Over the course of the past century all Americans, Black and White, have experienced improvements in health and longevity, in intelligence test scores, and in socioeconomic status. Moreover, the gap between Blacks and Whites has become more narrow in each of the areas mentioned, but our nation will face a serious challenge unless we begin to educate minority students more "equally with White students, particularly in the science-based fields" (Hamburg 1992, 298).

By the year 2020 nearly half of all school-age children will be non-White; in the 1990s minorities already were the majority of primary and secondary school students in twenty-three of the twenty-five largest cities (Hamburg 1992, 297). Census 2000 showed a total population of 281,426,906, a 13.2 percent increase over Census 1990. Blacks identifying as Black only increased by 4.7 million, or 15.6 percent since 1990, and adding those identifying as Black and at least one other race would bring the increase to 6.4 million, or a 21.5 percent increase. The total Black population is 36.4 million, or 12.9 percent of the U.S. total population. Census 2000 shows Hispanic or Latino population of 35.3 million, representing a 57.9 percent increase over 1990, close to parity with Black Americans, or 12.5 percent of the total U.S. population (U.S. Dept. of Commerce 2001). As I pointed out earlier, demographic projections are that the Black population as of the year 2030 will have doubled the 1990 figure and will be 62 million. If we do not develop the full potential of these young people, we will be inviting untold misery for the entire nation.

America's technologically educated workforce, Hamburg reminds us, has traditionally come from a small fraction of the population, about 6 percent, the "White, male, college-educated population," yet "the traditional white male source of scientists and engineers is inadequate." Our nation must accept the challenge of educating previously excluded minority groups and women, not only out of concerns for equity and fairness, but also to protect our "economic vitality, democratic civility, and military security." He mentions the sweeping changes in educational opportunity necessary to bring about more equal educational opportunity for minority groups, especially Blacks. These educational interventions should cover the entire life cycle from prenatal, postnatal, preschool, and school-age years, and into adulthood. Very young children especially without adequate supportive families, would require the equivalence of surrogate parenting. Schooling should cover a core curriculum meeting national standards and norms, with a longer school day, and year-round schooling involving parent-teacher community and church leadership and teamwork.

But education should also be combined with equalization of job opportunity, as Robert Solow has pointed out (1998). He argues that welfare as we know it must be changed, but not in the inadequate manner of the

1996 Welfare Reform Act. Solow maintains that simply putting people off
the welfare rolls without giving them jobs increases the unemployment
rate of the lowest-paid workers and may leave the children of young mothers with less developmental support. Jobs should be provided either in the
private sector or by the government, as well as high-quality child care for
working mothers. Roemer, agreeing with Solow and the others, points out
that genuine welfare reform should also include compensatory educational
opportunity for adults as well as school-age children, and that such a program would be very expensive. It would require at least 6.5 percent of the
nation's gross national product in contrast to the 2.4 percent currently
spent. Politicians favor welfare reform but do not support the increased
taxation it would demand. A guaranteed job would of course be a benefit
for all Americans, making it possible for all to have increased feelings of
self-respect, dignity, and the ability to become productive citizens.

Welfare reform should not only carry with it increased governmental
expenditures, it should also be obligatory that welfare recipients meet
standards of social functioning in areas of work, education, and civic responsibility. According to Lawrence Meade (1986, 1997), a political scien-
tist who has carefully analyzed this problem, even though this can fairly be
described as benign paternalism, which runs counter both to liberal and
conservative frames of mind, it is a federal policy more likely to advance
the integration of the so called "underclass" into mainstream American society. We must set standards but also make it possible for people to meet
them. I agree with Glenn Loury (1998) that a combination of increased
benefits along with increased responsibility would be not only productive
but well received by welfare recipients.

Welfare reform should also include programs to interrupt the cycle of
welfare dependence from one generation to the next. Daniels, Kennedy,
and Kawachi (1999) cite as one example the twenty-seven-year study of
a high-quality early childhood developmental program for children
three to five years old in a low-income neighborhood in Ypsilanti, Michigan (Schweinhart, Barnes, and Weikart 1993). Compared to a control
group, those in the intervention group had completed more schooling
by age twenty-seven and were more likely to be employed, to own a
home, and to be married with children. They also had experienced fewer
criminal problems and teenage pregnancies and were less likely to have
mental health problems.

Other demonstration programs with relatively low-intensity intervention have shown great promise. In one program, pregnant single teenage
mothers were visited once a month during pregnancy, and these monthly

visits continued until the children were two years old. During the ninety-minute interviews the visiting nurse followed a structured protocol covering such items as the developmental progress of the infant, advice on contraception and avoidance of subsequent pregnancy, advantages of involving the putative father and relatives, building a friendship support system, school completion and job training, and use of community health and social services. Fifteen years later, extensive follow-up showed considerably higher social function for these young mothers and their children. These findings clearly demonstrated more successful social functioning in comparison with a control group. This sample of predominantly White teenage mothers in Elmira County of upstate New York is currently being replicated with a 1990 sample of Black single mothers in Memphis who have been followed already for more than ten years with favorable results (Olds et al. 1997; Olds et al. 1998; Kitzman et al. 1997; Earls 1998; Loury 1998).

I believe that our nation will continue to equalize opportunity for all, and that the test case will be the measure of equality achieved by Black Americans. With their increasing numbers Blacks will become either more productive members of mainstream society or they will become progressively isolated, alienated, and forced into retaliatory and self-defeating behavior. As a nation we need them more as college graduates than as prisoners. It will probably cost much less, financially and in every other way, to choose greater opportunity rather than oppression.

EQUALIZING THE HEALTH STATUS OF BLACK AMERICANS

Byrd and Clayton (2000) have given us the most comprehensive history of race, medicine, and health care in the United States. What they refer to as the "Second Reconstruction in Black Health" lasted from 1965 to 1975, a part of the civil rights movement: desegregation of hospitals through court rulings, civil rights laws outlawing discrimination in government-funded health programs, the passage of Medicare and Medicaid, removing financial barriers to health care, neighborhood health centers in underserved communities, and affirmative action admission to medical school and postgraduate training. Within this ten-year period African American health improved by "every measure of health status, utilization and outcome." Stagnation occurred after 1975, and relative and/or absolute decline (compared to Whites) began after 1980. These improvements still left remaining a significant amount of race-based health disparities.

In November 2000 President Clinton signed into law legislation elevating the status of the Office of Research on Minority Health to that of a Center in the National Institutes of Health and provided 130 million dollars for the new center, nearly 40 million dollars a year more than previous funding. Additionally, Congress allocated funds for the Institute of Medicine to conduct a study on racial bias in medicine, which was scheduled to be completed in early 2002. A national task force has been set up to coordinate efforts of the Department of Human Services, the American Public Health Association, the AMA, and National Medical Association to bring about positive change in addition to study. There are indications that the initiative to remove racial health status disparities will be continued despite the change from Democratic to Republican leadership (Dirks 2001).

As David R. Williams and Toni D. Rucker (2000) point out, "Effectively addressing health care disparities will require comprehensive efforts by multiple sectors of society to address large inequities in major societal institutions," including "concerted societal-wide efforts to confront and eliminate discrimination in education, employment, housing, criminal justice and other areas of society which will improve the socioeconomic status . . . of disadvantaged minority populations and indirectly provide them greater access to medical care . . . as a fundamental right of citizenship" (33). It is my own opinion that chances are slim for a straightforward political commitment at federal, state, and local levels to equalize the health care or health status specifically for Blacks. As Clayton and Byrd (2001) state, extreme and persistent race-based health disparities exist because "public policy and funding have traditionally followed the concerns of the majority (White) population and not necessarily the public health problems of the nation's underserved and disenfranchised." They note that the mortality rate ratio is at least 1.5 times greater for Blacks than Whites in eight of the fifteen leading causes of death. These Black-White ratios lessened between 1989 and 1996 in some areas like homicide (from 6.6 to 6.2), kidney disease (3.1 to 2.6), chronic liver disease and cirrhosis (1.7 to 1.3), and cardiovascular disease (1.89 to 1.8). There was no improvement from 1989 to 1996 in the disease categories of cancer, a death ratio of 1.3, or pneumonia and influenza, which remained stable at 1.5. Deterioration or widening of mortality ratios from 1989 to 1996 were found in HIV-AIDS (from 3.3 to 5.8), septicemia (2.7 to 2.8), diabetes mellitus (2.3 to 2.4), heart disease (1.4 to 1.5), and perinatal conditions (2.3 to 2.4).

It should be apparent, from these movements and change, that a massive intervention would be required to eliminate these health status disparities. We should also note, however, that these same authors pointed out that during the decade of 1965 to 1975 the civil rights movement was accompanied by sweeping and overall improvements in the health of

Black Americans relative to Whites and relative to anything experienced earlier in American history. What strikes me as the crucial factor is that it was during that same 1965–75 decade that we experienced dramatic improvements in civil rights for women, an impressive war on poverty and actual reduction in numbers of impoverished Americans in general, and improved civil rights for the handicapped and other disadvantaged Americans. In my view major improvements for Blacks can occur only when there is simultaneous improvements for other constituencies. What are the prospects therefore for a revival of these positive social changes?

REFRAMING THE PROBLEM: AFFIRMATIVE ACTION FOR ALL AMERICANS

It is my opinion that as a nation we must become aware that we have a national health status problem, as well as problems in our delivery of the whole array of human services and a need to improve our general social welfare and health. In speeches of our national leaders, and in presentation by the media, the American public is kept continuously aware of our economic health as shown by such indicators as the gross domestic product, the stock market, the index of leading economic indicators, the balance of trade, the inflation rate, the consumer confidence level, and other such measures. All of these barometers tell us how we are doing economically, warn of the threat of economic downturn or recession, and give authority to the Federal Reserve to raise or lower interest rates to prevent serious damage to our economic welfare. Miringoff and Miringoff (1999) make the case that we need similar mechanisms to monitor, forecast, and modulate the social health of the nation. While we lead the world in monitoring our economy, we lag behind other developed nations in monitoring our social health. Beginning in the 1970s Great Britain and seventeen other industrialized nations have issued annual surveys focusing on health, housing, education, safety, employment, and access to services, stressing behavior and concrete experience of their citizenry rather than just documenting their opinion and attitudes. In this country, while we are relatively weak or inactive in reporting social indicators at the national level, many localities since the 1970s have established projects to monitor and report on the quality of community life. With major foundation support, the Miringoffs for the past twelve years have headed the Fordham Institute for Innovation in Social Policy, and have reported overall U.S. and state scores on an index of social health. In the period 1970–96 their indicators have shown positive and negative changes within our nation, how the states compare with each other and also how we perform relative to other nations.

For example in the 1970–96 period, four national indicators improved: infant mortality, high school dropouts, poverty for those over sixty-five years of age, and life expectancy for those over sixty-five. However, seven indicators showed worsening performance: child abuse, child poverty, teenage suicide, number of health care uninsured, average weekly wages, income inequality, and violent crime. Another six indicators showed variable performance: teenage drug use, teenage births, alcohol-related traffic fatalities, affordable housing, and employment. Our political leadership is not held accountable for the state of our social health, nor are we given by the media anything like a daily "weather report, a sports report, an economic report, a business report and a political report. What is missing . . . is the idea of a 'social report'" (Miringoff and Miringoff 1999, 172). Miringoff and Miringoff go on to say that "in a democracy, problems generally are not addressed until they are recognized and understood by the public. Yet many social conditions have worsened for a generation without significant public knowledge."

Even less is the public aware of how unfavorably our social health compares with other nations. Our unemployment rate was in 1996 good, the second lowest of the ten nations with acceptable data, but we had the highest rate of child poverty among Western industrialized nations, ranking seventeenth of seventeen; we were eighteenth out of eighteen on income inequality, and near the bottom of the list in indicators such as elderly poverty, high school dropouts, infant mortality, life expectancy, teenage births, wages, youth homicide, and youth suicide. Raphael (2000) points out that despite spending a greater percentage of gross domestic product, 13.5 percent, on health care than any other industrialized nation, "for nearly all available outcome measures, the United States ranked near the bottom of the OECD countries in 1996 and the rate of improvement for most of the indicators has been slower than the median OECD Country. . . . Among the 29 Organization for Economic Corporation and Development nations, USA life expectancy ranked nineteenth for females and twenty-second for males" (404).

While there is a need to develop and implement programs to bring Black Americans up to an acceptable standard of health, we should accept the challenge to do the same for all Americans. Raphael (2000), in a review of the emerging literature on the social determinants of health, maintains that it is the growing economic inequality within the United States that affects health directly by creating greater poverty and indirectly by weakening communal social structures that support social and health services, and by decreasing social cohesion and civil commitment (427).

While it is true that health differences in the United States are related to race, this obscures the fact that even larger differences are related to levels of income class, which receives relatively little attention. Low-income American families "are at a distinct disadvantage compared with similarly situated families in other nations" (406). Beyond a consideration of the importance of lifestyle and community support structures in protecting health, a greater focus is required on such basic economic factors as the effects of globalization on labor demand and changes in tax structure and funding of social welfare programs in the United States. In other words, there are fundamental limitations to addressing racial and ethnic health inequalities rather than our national health status by comparison with other developed nations.

Starfield (2000) notes that the United States ranks twelfth among a group of thirteen of the most developed nations on health indices covering the life cycle from infancy through the elderly years. Removing U.S. Blacks from our national health statistics does not improve our cross-national comparative rank. In the United States those states with the most unequal income distributions "invest less in public education, have larger uninsured populations, and spend less on safety nets. . . . Even when controlling for median income, income inequality explains about 40 percent of the between-state variation in the percentage of children in the fourth grade who fall below the basic reading level. Similarly, strong associations are seen in the percentage of high school dropout rates" (Daniels, Kennedy, and Kawachi 1999, 223).

Daniels, Kennedy, and Kawachi (1999) conclude that we should consider such disparities "inequalities when they are avoidable, unnecessary, and unfair" (225). When age, gender, race, and ethnic differences in health status exist that are "independent of socioeconomic differences," they "raise distinct questions about equity of justice." Following John Rawls (1971), these authors conclude that health inequities cannot be overcome except by paying attention to the primary social goods all persons require in addition to health care, including "liberty, powers, opportunities, income and wealth, and the social bases of self-respect" (229).

There are two ways to address the issue of how compensation should be made to Black Americans for unpaid labor during almost 250 years of chattel slavery, and their subsequent exclusion from asset-building governmental policies that were made available to Whites. Randall Robinson (2000) has been joined by other prominent Black lawyers who have filed suit against the U.S. government and several corporations to win financial reparations to make up for assets that should be restored to Black people here. It is Robinson's position that this is a claim that should be made even if the chance for success is slim, because it is the right thing to do, especially since we live under an adversarial system of justice and should use any legal means to correct this long-standing injustice. In my view there is a basic flaw in the argument for reparations: slavery was immoral indeed, but it was legal and governmentally protected. Moreover the institution of slavery not only impoverished Blacks, it diminished and stunted the development of our nation as a whole in ways that still survive in our American way of life. Both Black and White Americans should be freed from this hand of the dead past.

Another and better approach to achieve compensation for many generations of unpaid labor was proposed by Martin Luther King in *Why We Can't Wait* (1963). It has been a general government policy to reward veterans returning from war with benefits they might have lost during years of service, such as the GI Bill of Rights following World War II. Benefits included subsidies to finance their continued education, extra points on civil service examinations, lower interest rates to purchase a home or to launch a business, medical care and long-term financial grants if they had suffered physical or emotional disability. King believed that, while no amount of money could adequately pay for the many years of exploitation and humiliation during slavery, there is a long tradition in common law that remedy should be made when human beings have been financially damaged. He thought this country should launch a broad-based "Bill of Rights for the Disadvantaged," patterned on the GI Bill of Rights. However, King believed this massive social transfer should be paid not only to Blacks but also to poor Whites, especially in the South, because their poverty largely resulted from the fact that their labor "was cheapened by the involuntary servitude of the Black man" (1963, 138). He went on to say that White workers even now are pacified by being allowed to feel superior and thereby distanced from Black workers.

The nation would have much to gain by a determined effort to eliminate poverty, especially, and of the highest priority, to eliminate child poverty. During the past generation, Americans, Black and White, have experienced a breakdown of the two-parent family: in 1950 only 17 percent of Blacks and 5 percent of Whites lived in households headed by women, but in 1990 we had 56 percent of Blacks and 17 percent of Whites with absent fathers. Hacker points out also that the 9.9:1 ratio of the rate of unmarried Black mothers to unmarried White mothers in 1950 (16.8 percent Black to 1.7 percent White), was reduced in 1988 to a ratio of 4.3 to 1 because the increase for White women was greater than that for Blacks (1992, 74).

Hambroke et al. (1996, 180–81) point out that in 1993 the proportion in poverty of young children of White single-parent mothers, (43 percent), is "about the same as had already been reached by Black single-parent mothers in the late 1960s" (184). Forces producing poverty are not static but rather a dynamic system: "some groups in society are more vulnerable to these escalating forces, others less so, but all are moving in the same direction" (184). A family is said to be in a state of deep poverty if their family income is 50 percent below the poverty line—only half of what a family needs for basic expenses like food, housing and other living costs. The percentage of White children under age six in deep poverty in 1993 was 7.7 percent, whereas for Black children under age six, about 33 percent live in deep poverty. "Over the past two decades, the percentage of children living in such deep poverty has more than doubled, from 1.1 million in 1975 to 2.8 million in 1994. Forty-seven percent of all young children are in poverty as compared with a third, 32 percent, in 1975, just before the rapid decline in economic growth" (181). We should bear in mind that although the percentages of Black children are more than four times higher, the actual numbers of White children living in deep poverty, exceeds the Black number: of the 17.1 million children in the United States who are under six years of age, 80 percent are White, 16 percent Black.

While it is true in my opinion that disparities between Blacks and Whites in the field of health should be identified and monitored and that special efforts should be launched to remove them, it should be kept in mind that since the 1960s we have not heard a call for our nation to renew a general war on poverty. White poverty remains essentially invisible. There has been a largely successful political strategy of labeling increased federal governmental spending for human services as a plan to advance the cause of African Americans at the expense of the White middle-class taxpayers. As Klinker and Smith summarize the present situation: the greatest impediments to greater social and ethnic equality are to be found in the resurgence of arguments for state and local governments instead of national government initiatives, increased calls for "color blind" governmental action, of personal initiatives as solutions, resurgent "scientific racism" such as the Bell curve propaganda, decline in civil rights law enforcement, and diminished enthusiasm for a racially integrated nation. On the other hand, there are strong forces to continue genuine removal of ethnic disparities, such as support for civil rights law enforcement and for ending racial profiling, and a beginning awareness that economic inequality is a major threat to our cohesion as a national community. Klinker and Smith also believe that specific means must be found to reform the criminal justice system, which has devastated so many young Black men. Another positive force would be the reinstitution of the military draft on an egalitarian basis, to require all young Americans of different racial, ethnic, and social class backgrounds to learn to work with, and to develop friendships with, persons of different backgrounds.

A HOPEFUL FORECAST

Robert W. Fogel, the 1993 Nobel Prize winner in economics, believes it is altogether feasible that inequality nationally and worldwide be reduced over the long term. The record of the twentieth century "contrasts sharply with that of the two preceding centuries. In every measure that we have bearings on the standard of living, such as real income, homelessness, life expectancy, and height, the gains of the lower classes have been greater than those experienced by the population as a whole, whose overall standard of living has also improved" (2000, 143). Economists use the Gini ratio to measure income inequality (zero is perfect equality and 1.0 represents maximum inequality). Data for England is available to show that the Gini ratio was 0.65 near the beginning of the eighteenth century, 0.55 beginning the twentieth century, and 0.32 in 1973, when it bottomed out in England and "also in the United States and other rich nations" (143).

A striking example is shown by life expectancy improvement: in 1875 the British upper class lived seventeen years longer than the population as a whole. Today, the "advantage of the richest classes over the poorest is only about two years. Thus, about seven-eighths of the social gap in longevity has disappeared." Longevity for the lower classes went from forty-one years at birth in 1875 to seventy-five years today—and again there are roughly comparable figures for the United States. "Indeed, there has been a larger increase in life expectancy during the past century than there was during the previous 200,000 years. If anything sets our century apart from the past, it is this huge increase in the longevity of the lower classes" (Fogel 2000, 143).

Average height and weight, which are measures of improving nutrition, have shown similar changes. Reductions in homelessness tell a similar story of improvement over the long term, but the United States in recent decades has seen an increase of homelessness among the most vulnerable segments of our population: mentally ill persons released from hospitals to communities with inadequately funded programs to meet their needs; other homeless people are "chronically poor, young, and inadequately trained for the current job market" (Fogel 2000, 145).

However, Fogel notes that despite the sharp rise in incomes, "especially at the low end of the income distribution, the moral crisis of the cities remains unresolved . . . such problems as drug addiction, alcoholism, births to unmarried teenage girls, rape, the battery of women and children, broken families, violent teenage death, and crime are generally more severe today than they were a century ago" (172).

Fogel is convinced that simply gaining more income or possessions does not automatically increase morality, virtue, or spiritual growth, as can be seen in current observation of all social classes. When he speaks of the severe maldistribution of spiritual resources, he is not referring to formal religious or church membership but rather to such psychological resources as self-realization (a feeling of developing one's full potential as a person), a sense of purpose, a vision of opportunity, a sense of the mainstream of work and life, a strong family ethic, a capacity to engage with diverse groups, a work ethic, a sense of discipline, self-esteem (2000, 204–5). In the United States, as in other rich countries, overeating is a greater problem than undereating. The "opportunities to fulfill one's potential are more unequally distributed than food, consumer durables, or health care" (178).

Fogel is optimistic that the next six decades will see further reductions in the unequal distributions of both material and spiritual resources, fueled by such factors as the pressure for improved educational attainment, the world demand for more skills and professional manpower, and increasing political power of ethnic minorities and women (2000, 238). However he anticipates resistance to the development of a smooth transition from "a governing minority that is predominatly White and Protestant to a governing majority that is nonwhite and nonProtestant, one that does not sacrifice fundamental egalitarian ethical, political, social, and economic principles" (239–40).

SUMMARY

My concluding opinion is that affirmative action at all levels of education, from preschool through university, represents the best policy and program to build a strong, single, and ethnically integrated nation. As others have pointed out, these past thirty years of affirmative action admissions to the most prestigious colleges, universities, and professional schools have produced a strong African American middle class that is providing leadership not only for Black people but for the benefit of all Americans. Nothing of this magnitude has been done in this country since Reconstruction following the Civil War, when an abortive effort was made to enforce the Thirteenth, Fourteenth, and Fifteenth Amendments to our constitution, which were designed to abolish slavery for the benefit of all of our people.

A major reason for my optimism about the future of affirmative action in higher education comes from the report in the *Journal of Blacks in Higher Education* ("Progress of Black Student Matriculations" 1999), which shows that the major universities in the South are firmly behind these programs. Among the nation's twenty-seven highest-ranked universities and twenty-nine highest-ranked liberal arts colleges, the University of North Carolina at Chapel Hill for the second year in a row had the highest percentage of Black freshmen in the entering class (412, or 12.1 percent), the same as in the previous year. This is more than triple the rate at Notre Dame, Berkeley, Carnegie Mellon, and the University of Chicago. In fact "the four top-tier schools with the highest percentage of Black freshmen are all in the South" The University of Virginia, Duke University, and Emory University all had more than 9.0 percent. The University of Virginia (which was built by slave craftsmen, but which admitted its first Black student only in 1959), was in second place at 10 percent, down from 11.1 percent the previous year. Virginia had been in first place for five years from 1993 to 1997. The premier universities in the South are now enrolling the most talented Blacks, who earlier had been forced to enroll in the segregated state-funded universities in their states. Quite clearly the South has now joined all other major university centers in our land in providing first-class education to all citizens. In 1997 the 105 historically Black colleges and universities enrolled only 16 percent of all Black college students (*New York Public Library* 1999, 176). In 1970 they enrolled 58 percent (Willie and Edmonds 1978, 92), and in that same year the overwhelming majority of Black college graduates had gone to those schools. Christopher Lucas (1994) in his *American Higher Education: A History* comments on this significant desegregation of American higher education for Blacks: "By 1987, for the first time in American history, black students were more likely to matriculate at predominantly White institutions than at traditionally black schools. Slightly less than one in every five black students was then enrolled at a black college" (247). He goes on to state that advocates of Black institutions are not agreed that this is all favorable, pointing out that 40 percent of the Blacks are enrolled in two-year institutions and might be better served by going to a Black college, 90 percent of which are four-year schools. They claim also that Black schools probably have a better success rate in graduating high-risk students, and in providing a generally more comfortable social life.

My own view is that students should choose the college or university they prefer but that great weight should be given to the advantages of receiving an education in an environment where everyone does not look, behave, and think as you do. Particularly this is true as we become increasingly members of a world community. It is a positive gain for our nation that as we advance into the twenty-first century our Black and White middle-class leadership will have been educated in the same colleges and universities, giving them a foundational experience as they create "one nation indivisible with liberty and justice for all."

Affirmative action to eliminate racial disparities in the health status of Blacks will require a fundamental change in our frame of reference, including a commitment to improve the health of all of our citizens who live in poverty. Even the health status of more affluent Americans does not compare favorably with other developed nations.

EPILOGUE

In the more than fifty years since my graduation from the University of Michigan Medical School in 1946, as the only African American among the 145 graduates, I have been both an eyewitness to and an active player in the changing role of Blacks in American medicine.

When I graduated, I was advised that I could choose my internship and subsequent postgraduate appointments from among no more than half a dozen hospitals. Half of them had almost all Black patients, and the others were general public charity hospitals serving low-income populations. It was only a few years later that increasing fractions of medical school graduates began to pursue additional years of residency training to become specialists. The medical world in those years was segregated by race and income, though this system was beginning to change with the end of World War II.

In 1946 the huge Wayne County General Hospital accepted me and another graduate from Meharry Medical College as its first Black interns. At the end of that year, during which we were well received both by patients and the hospital staff, we were stunned to find that we had not been invited to attend the staff Christmas party. One of the other interns, a White physician who had graduated from a southern medical school, told me that he and several others had argued that we should be invited. Having lost that argument on a vote, he wanted to make a gift to me if I would accept it. His father, the owner of a clothing store, had sent him two suits; he and I wore the same size, and he wanted to give one of the suits to me. I accepted, assuring him that he was not indebted to me because of the party. This incident taught me a personal lesson: young professionals, beginning a year as Blacks and Whites, could at the end of that year recognize each other as persons—as persons who see and renounce the intimate cruelty of race prejudice.

Another powerful experience occurred in the 1950s, when I was developing a private practice toward the end of my training. My first office was in our home in Brooklyn, an attractive brownstone that had been the home and office of a White psychiatrist who was moving out of the neighborhood because it was rapidly becoming all Black. One of my White instructors, who supervised my psychotherapy cases, thought highly of my work and referred a young White schoolteacher to me. She had been sent to him by an internist who thought her psychosomatic problems might respond to therapy. She came to see me several times but then terminated. The internist, it turned out, had learned that the patient was being treated by a Black psychiatrist in a Black neighborhood, and denounced my instructor for sending the patient to me.

My instructor and I reviewed the situation in great detail and came to one important conclusion—I should relocate my office to downtown Brooklyn Heights, where most of the specialists practiced. Both Black and White patients would be comfortable on visits to me at such a site. Being accepted into one of those office buildings was a tortured process, but the fifth landlord or business manager I approached rented me an attractive office. By happenstance his firm managed the real estate properties of one of Brooklyn's largest Black churches.

As the next few years unfolded, my practice flourished. My patients were about evenly divided between Blacks and Whites, and I received referrals from my professional associates and personal friends, who were also about evenly divided between the two races. A number of my patients were family members of my White colleagues, who referred them to me for care. Contrast this with another story. A friend of mine, a White specialist in internal medicine, had for some years taken care of a prominent Black businessman who was plunged into a deep depression after his son committed suicide. The internist wanted to refer him to me, but the patient refused. He insisted on being referred to a White psychiatrist. My reaction to this is—you win some and you lose some. For the best treatment result, the patient must make the choice. But many of the Black middle class must overcome their view that Black specialists are second-rate. There is room for new learning all around.

My first year at Cornell, 1968, was in many ways a pivotal one. I had been selected by a search committee that consisted of two senior faculty members, who were convinced that Cornell should join other leading schools in developing an affirmative action admissions program, and three White medical students, who were quite generally activist in favor of affirmative action and against the Vietnam War. My career interests and activities convinced them that I was a good choice. Since, however, there was only one Black faculty member on the full-time salaried faculty, and her interests were primarily in research, and only two Black students from

Africa, I did not have much of a support system. Once a week a faculty member and I were joined by two other Black internists on the Cornell Voluntary Faculty who also had admitting privileges at the New York Hospital. Our meetings were an important source of friendly emotional support and general information.

The summer research program I designed required twenty very able minority students to be with us at the medical center for ten weeks following their junior year of college. Each student would work half time on the research project of a faculty member; in the other half of their time we provided them background information on the health care delivery system as it related to the health problems of minority communities. As the first year developed, I was given my own background briefing on potential friends within the medical school community. For the entire year I had lunch once a week with the three medical students who had been on the search committee. The two faculty members who had been on the search committee met with me almost as often. The selection of faculty sponsors was no problem, and my formal and informal support system rapidly expanded. It is of some interest to me that one of the three students from that original search committee went on to become a psychiatrist and is now chairman of the psychiatry department in one of the nation's leading medical schools.

During my eleven years at Cornell I felt great pride in helping produce the first large cohort of minority medical school graduates, who would become a part of the mainstream of medicine in this country. By 1980, when I left the school, I was convinced that only a long-term study of the career development of a large sample of minority graduates, compared with an equal number of their nonminority classmates, would establish how much difference they were making in the racial integration of American medicine. No longer were 85 percent of Black physicians coming from Howard and Meharry; now 85 percent were graduating from all the other U.S. medical schools. Thirty years later, with that study having been undertaken, we can see how much of a difference these physicians are making in the lives of many people.

Heading the psychiatry department at Harlem Hospital Center in 1982 was a decision I reached on feeling a need to be more fully involved in the changing field of psychiatry. Harlem Hospital at the time was a thirteen-hundred-bed general hospital with the full spectrum of medical and surgical specialties, located in central Harlem's population of 250,000, more than 90 percent Black. For five years the psychiatry search committee had been unable to select a candidate acceptable to Columbia University, which held the affiliate contract to hire and supervise all physician staff, to the city's Health and Hospitals Corporation, which hired all other staff and financed the Columbia affiliation contract, and to members of the Harlem community. As a municipal hospital, Harlem Hospital Center always depended on support from the mayor, Harlem's political leaders and general community, and labor unions. The psychiatry residency training program had progressively weakened. My decision to accept the challenge to go to Harlem came from a belief that out of my experiences, background, training, and friendships within the medical establishment, I could develop a strong set of mental health services for the central Harlem community. Shortly after my appointment the psychiatry department grew from thirty-two to sixty-eight inpatient beds, with a large ambulatory service for all age groups. It accepted responsibility for staffing and running the drug treatment programs previously supervised by an ambulatory treatment service.

In time Harlem provided me with greater understanding of how the medical system works. On my retirement at the end of 1999 the hospital had shrunk down to 230 beds. With downsizing of patient care, all residency training programs became smaller; the psychiatry program, which had had thirty-five slots, was cut in half. A lack of political and community support, and the advent of managed care, threatened the hospital's survival. I learned that even though Harlem Hospital Center was on the surface a Black hospital, in reality it was not significantly controlled by Blacks. City and university politics, even more than labor union politics, made it impossible for the hospital leadership and community to carry out a relevant medical mission with sustained financial support.

As patients leave the municipal hospital system, seeking care in the private voluntary sector, it is quite possible that this shrinking of Harlem Center Hospital is for the best. As minority physicians leave the municipal hospital system, greater numbers move onto the staff of major university teaching hospitals. During my nearly twenty years at Harlem our large psychiatry residency training program only trained about four Black graduates from U.S. medical schools. While more than half of the five hundred we trained were Black physicians, they came from the Caribbean or from Africa. Most of the other trainees were from Third World countries. Medical and surgical residency training programs at Harlem experienced the same trend. In the 1970s large numbers of U.S. medical school minority graduates selected Harlem Hospital Center for postgraduate training, but this was no longer the case in the 1980s and 1990s. Where are they now going for training? To the major teaching hospitals around the nation.

As we have seen in the thirty-year progress report on affirmative action at Cornell, the medical school's minority graduates uniformly are placed in prestigious training programs. At Cornell there are currently forty-three fully salaried minority faculty, compared with one in 1970. This is an indication that affirmative action works, and that Blacks and other minority physicians are becoming securely included in American medicine.

"Advancing Minority Student Recruitment." 1996. *Cornell Medicine* 1:18–21.

Allen, W. R., and J. O. Jewell. 1995. "African American Education since *An American Dilemma.*" *Daedalus* 124:77–100.

American Medical Association (AMA). 1976a. *Directory of Accredited Residencies, 1975–76.* Annual Report on Graduate Medical Education in the United States. Chicago: AMA Publications.

———. 1976b. "Medical Education in the United States, 1975–76" (76th Annual Report). *Journal of the American Medical Association* 236:2984.

———. 1977. *Directory of Accredited Residencies, 1977–78.* Annual Report on Graduate Medical Education in the United States. Chicago: American Medical Association Publications.

———. 1994. *American Medical Directory.* 34th ed. Chicago: AMA Publications.

"Annual Report (Eightieth): Medical Education in the United States 1979–80." 1980. *Journal of the American Medical Association* 244 (5).

Association of American Medical Colleges (AAMC). 1968. Proceedings for 1968. *Journal of Medical Education* 44:349.

———. 1970. *Report of the Task Force of the Association of American Medical Colleges to the Inter-Association Committee on Expanding Educational Opportunities in Medicine for Blacks and Other Minority Students.* Washington, D.C.: AAMC Publications.

———. 1976. Brief as amicus curiae. *Regents of the University of California v. Bakke,* 438 U.S. 265 (1978), 1–20.

———. 1977. *Medical School Admission Requirements, 1978–1979, United States and Canada.* Washington, D.C.: AAMC.

———. 1978. *Report of the AAMC's Task Force on Minority Student Opportunities in Medicine.* Washington, D.C.: AAMC.

———. 1980. *Graduate Medical Education: Proposals for the Eighties.* Washington, D.C.: AAMC.

———. 1982–83. *Minority Student Opportunities in United States Medical Schools.* Washington, D.C.: AAMC.

———. 1988. *Minority Student Opportunities in the United States Medical Schools.* 14th ed. Washington, D.C.: AAMC.

———. 1998. *Minority Students in Medical Education: Facts and Figures XI.* Washington, D.C.: Office of Community and Minority Programs, AAMC.

————. 2000. *Minority Student Opportunities in United States Medical Schools.* 15th ed. Washington, D.C.: AAMC.

Ayres, I. 1991. "Driving: Gender and Race Discrimination in Retail Car Negotiations." *Harvard Law Review* 104:817–72.

Bergeison, L., and J. C. Cantor. 1999. "The Minority Medical Education Program." In *To Improve Health and Health Care 2000,* ed. S. Isaacs and J. R. Knickman, 41–61. San Francisco: Jossey-Bass.

Bowen, W. G., and D. Bok. 1998. *The Shape of the River: Long-Term Consequences of Considering Race in College and University Admissions.* Princeton: Princeton University Press.

Brief for Petitioner. 1976. *Regents of the University of California v. Bakke,* 438 U.S. 265 (1978), 1–87.

Bundy, M. 1977. "The Issue before the Court: Who Gets Ahead in America." *Atlantic Monthly,* November 1977, 41–54.

Burke, Y. B. 1977. "Minority Admissions to Medical Schools: Problems and Opportunities." *Journal of Medical Education* 52:731–38.

Byrd, W. M., and L. A. Clayton. 2000a. *An American Health Dilemma.* Vol. 1: *A Medical History of African Americans and the Problem of Race: Beginnings to 1900.* New York: Routledge.

————. 2000b. "Race, Medicine, and Health Care in the United States: A Historical Survey." *Journal of the National Medical Association* 93 (Supplement): 115–345, 355–545.

Cantor, J. C., L. Bergeison, and L. C. Baker. 1998. "Effect of an Intensive Education Program for Minority College Students and Recent Graduates." *Journal of the American Medical Association* 280:772–76.

Cantor, J. C., E. L. Miles, L. C. Baker, and D. C. Barker. 1996. "Physician Services to the Underserved: Implications for Affirmative Action in Medical Education." *Inquiry* 33:157–80.

Canty, D. 1969. *A Simple Society: Alternatives to Urban Apartheid.* New York: Praeger.

Carnegie Council on Policy Studies in Higher Education. 1977. *Selective Admissions in Higher Education.* San Francisco: Jossey-Bass.

Carson, B., with C. Murphy. 1990. *Gifted Hands.* Grand Rapids, Mich.: Zondervan Books.

Ceci, S. J. 1996. "American Education: Looking Inward and Outward." In *The State of Americans: This Generation and the Next,* ed. U. Bronfenbrenner et al., 185–207. New York: Free Press.

Clayton, L. A., and W. M. Byrd. 2001. "Race: A Major Health Status and Outcome Variable, 1980–1999." *Journal of the National Medical Association* 93:405.

"The Closing of Philadelphia General Hospital." 1978. *Urban Health* 7:40–47.

Cobb, M. 1964. "Integration of Hospitals." *Journal of the National Medical Association* 56:282–85, 287.

Cogan, L. 1968. *Negroes for Medicine: Report of a Macy Conference.* Baltimore: Johns Hopkins University Press.

Collins, K., K. Tenny, and D. Hughes. 2002. *Quality of Health Care for African Americans.* The Commonwealth Fund 2001 Health Care Survey. May. New York: Commonwealth Fund. www.cmwf.org.

Commission on Public General Hospitals. 1978. *The Future of the Public General Hospital: An Agenda for Transition.* Chicago: Hospital Research and Educational Trust.

Committee on Quality of Health Care in America. Institute of Medicine. 2001. *Crossing the Quality Chasm: A New Health System for the Twenty-First Century.* Washington, D.C.: National Academy Press.

Cornely, P. B. 1976. "Racism: The Ever Present Hidden Barrier to Health in Our Society." *American Journal of Public Health* 66:246–47.

Corwin, E. H., and G. E. Sturges. 1936. *Opportunities for the Medical Education of Negroes.* New York: Charles Scribner's Sons.

Crocker, A. R. 1975. *Characteristics of Black Physicians in the United States: Findings from a Survey.* Bureau of Health Resources Development, Public Health Service, DHEW Report No 75-147. Washington, D.C.: U.S. Government Printing Office.

Crosby, F., and C. VanDeVeer, eds. 2000. *Sex, Race, and Merit: Debating Affirmative Action in Education and Employment.* Ann Arbor: University of Michigan Press.

Cross, T. 1984. *The Black Power Imperative: Racial Inequality and the Politics of Non-Violence.* New York: Faulkner.

Cross, T., and R. B. Slater. 2000. "The Alarming Decline in the Academic Performance of African-American Men." *Journal Blacks in Higher Education* 27:82–87.

Cuca, J. M. 1977. *Career Choices of the 1976 Graduates of U.S. Medical Schools.* Washington, D.C.: Association of American Medical Colleges.

Curtis, J. 1971. *Blacks, Medical Schools, and Society.* Ann Arbor: University of Michigan Press.

———. 1975. "Minority Student Success and Failure with the National Intern and Resident Matching Program." *Journal of Medical Education* 50:563–70.

Dahlgren, G., and M. Whitehead. 1999. "Policies and Strategies to Promote Social Equity in Health." *Monitoring Equity in Health,* ed. Paula Braveman. Geneva: World Health Organization.

Daniels, N., B. P. Kennedy, and I. Kawachi. 1999. "Why Justice Is Good for Our Health: The Social Determinants of Health Inequalities." *Daedalus* 128: 215–51.

Davidson, R. O., and E. L. Lewis. 1997. "Affirmative Action and Other Special Consideration Admissions at the University of California at Davis, School of Medicine." *Journal of the American Medical Association* 278:1153–58.

Davis, B. 1976. "Sounding Board: Academic Standards in Medical Schools." *New England Journal of Medicine* 294:1118–19.

deVise, P. 1973. "Physician Migration from Island to Coastal States: Antipodal Examples of Illinois and California." *Journal of Medical Education* 48:141–51.

Dirks, D. P. 2001. "National Center for Minority Health Established: Changing of the Guard." *Minority Health Today* 2:48–49.

Division of Community and Minority Programs, Association of American Medical Colleges. 1996. *Project 3000 by 2000.* Washington, D.C.: AAMC.

Drake, S. 1971. "The Black University in the American Social Order: The Future of the Black Colleges." *Daedalus* 100:833–97.

Dreyfuss, J., and C. Lawrence. 1979. *The Bakke Case: The Politics of Inequality.* New York: Harcourt Brace Jovanovich.

Dworkin, R. 1998. "Affirming Affirmative Action." *New York Review of Books,* October 22, 91–102.

Earls, F. 1998. "Effects of Prenatal and Early Childhood Interventions." *Journal of the American Medical Association* 280:1271–72.

Fernandes, D. R., and P. J. Imperato. 1980. "Student Views of the Community Served by an Inner City Medical Center." *Journal of Medical Education* 55:751–57.

Fiscella, K., P. Franks, M. Gold, and C. Clancy. 2000. "Inequality in Quality: Addressing Socioeconomic, Racial, and Ethnic Disparities in Health Care." *Journal of the American Medical Association* 283:2579–84.

Fleming, J. E., G. R. Gill, and D. Swinton. 1978. *The Case for Affirmative Action for Blacks in Higher Education.* Washington, D.C.: Howard University Press.

Fogel, R. W. 1989. *Without Consent or Contract: The Rise and Fall of American Slavery.* New York: Norton.

———. 2000. *The Fourth Great Awakening and the Future of Egalitarianism.* Chicago: University of Chicago Press.

Fogel, R. W., and S. Engerman. 1974. *Time on the Cross: The Economics of American Negro Slavery.* Boston: Little, Brown.

Freeman, H., and R. Payne. 2000. "Racial Injustice in Health Care." *New England Journal of Medicine* 342:1045–47.

Fuchs, V. R. 1998. *Who Shall Live? Health, Economics, and Social Choice.* Rev. ed. River Edge, N.J.: World Scientific Press.

Gamble, V. N. 1995. *Making a Place for Ourselves: The Black Hospital Movement, 1920–1945.* New York-Oxford: Oxford University Press.

Ginzberg, E., M. Millman, and C. Brecher. 1979. "The Problematic Future of Public General Hospitals." *Health and Medical Care Services Review* 2(2).

Glazer, N. 1999. "Should the SAT Account for Race? Yes." *New Republic,* September 27, 26–29.

———. 1993. "A Tale of Two Cities." *New Republic,* August 2, 39–41.

Gordon, T. L., and D. G. Johnson. 1977. "Study of U.S. Medical School Applicants, 1975–76." *Journal of Medical Education* 52:707–30.

Graettinger, J. S. 1978. "Results of the NIRMP for 1977." *Journal of Medical Education* 53:96–102.

Gray, L. C. 1977. "The Geographic and Functional Distribution of Black Physicians: Some Research and Policy Considerations." *American Journal of Public Health* 67:519–26.

Grimshaw, A. D., ed. 1969. *Racial Violence in the United States.* Chicago: Aldine.

Hacker, A. 1992. *Two Nations: Black and White, Separate, Hostile, Unequal.* New York: Charles Scribner's Sons,

Hambroke, H., P. A. Morris, U. Bronfenbrenner, P. McClelland, E. Wethington, P. Moen, and S. J. Ceci. 1996. *Poverty and the Next Generation in the State of Americans.* New York: Free Press.

Hamburg, D. 1992. *Today's Children: Creating a Future Generation in Crisis.* New York: Random House.

The Handbook of Historically Black Colleges and Universities. 3d ed. 1999. Wilmington, Del.: Jireh and Associates.

Haynes, N. A. 1969. "The Distribution of Black Physicians in the U.S." *Journal of the American Medical Association* 210:93–95.

"Health and Science: A Study in Black and White." 2000. *American Medical News,* May 1, 22–23.

"Health Care in Newark." 1978. *Urban Health* 7:6–38.

"Health Care in Newark." 1979. *Urban Health* 8:42–45.

Higgins, Elizabeth J. 1979. *Comparison of Characteristics of U.S. Medical School Salaried Faculty in the Past Decade.* Washington, D.C.: AAMC, Division of Operational Studies.

"Historic Partnership Is First of Its Kind: APHA, HHS Join Forces to Combat Health Disparities." 2000. *Nation's Health* (American Public Health Association), May, pp. 1, 13.

Hochschild, J. L. 1995. *Facing Up to the American Dream: Race, Class, and the Soul of the Nation.* Princeton: Princeton University Press.

Hoffman, F. L. 1896. *Race Traits and Tendencies of the American Negro.* New York: Macmillan.

Holzer H., and D. Neumark. 2000. "Assessing Affirmative Action." *Journal of Economic Literature* 38:483–568.

"Homer G. Phillips Hospital: A Historic Hospital Faces Closing." 1976. *Urban Health* 5:22–27.

Iler, E., and M. Slater. 1998. "The Gateway Program: Ten-Year Lessons about Outcomes and Admissions Measures." *Academic Medicine* 73:1169–71.

Institute for the Study of Educational Policy, Howard University. 1976. *Equal Opportunity for Blacks in U.S. Higher Education: An Assessment.* Washington, D.C.: Howard University Press.

Jaynes, G. D., and R. M. Williams, eds. 1989. *A Common Destiny: Blacks and American Society.* Washington, D.C.: National Academy Press.

Johnson, D. G., and E. B. Hutchins. 1966. "Doctor or Dropout?" *Journal of Medical Education* 44:1099–1292.

Johnson, D. G., V. Smith, and S. Tarnoff. 1975. "Recruitment and Progress of Minority Medical School Entrants, 1970–1972." *Journal of Medical Education* 50:711–55.

Johnson, L. 1967. "History of the Education of Negro Physicians." *Journal of Medical Education* 42:432–41.

Johnson, L. J. 1998. "Minorities in Medical School and National Medical Fellowships, Inc.: Fifty Years and Counting." *Academic Medicine* 73:1044–51.

Jones, J. H. 1981. *Bad Blood: The Tuskegee Syphilis Experiment.* New York: The Free Press.

Jones S., and G. Weatherby. 1978. "Financing the Black College." In *Black Colleges in America,* ed. C. Willie and R. Edmonds. New York: Teachers' College Press.

JRB Associates. 1979. *Impact of the Closing of Philadelphia General Hospital.* Philadelphia: Fellowship Commission.

Kaiser Family Foundation. 2002. *National Survey of Physicians Part I: Doctors on Disparities in Medical Care—Highlights and Chartpack.* March. Menlo Park, Calif.: Henry J. Kaiser Family Foundation. www.kf.org.

Keith, S. N, R. M. Bell, and A. P. Williams. 1987. *Assessing the Outcome of Affirmative Action in Medical Schools: A Study of the Class of 1975.* Santa Monica, Calif.: Rand Corporation.

King, M. L., Jr. 1963. *Why We Can't Wait.* New York: Signet.

Kitzman, H., D. Olds, C. Henderson, et al. 1997. "Effects of Prenatal and Infancy Home Visitation by Nurses on Pregnancy Outcomes, Childhood Injuries, and Repeated Childbearing." *Journal of the American Medical Association* 276:644–52.

Klinker, P., and R. Smith. 1999. *The Unsteady March: The Rise and Decline of Racial Equality in America.* Chicago: University of Chicago Press.

Kluger, R. 1976. *Simple Justice: The History of Brown v. Board of Education and Black America's Struggle for Equality.* New York: Knopf.

Koleda, M., and J. Craig. 1976. "Minority Physician Practice, Interns, and Access to Health Care Services." *Looking Ahead and Projection Highlights,* vol. 2. National Planning Association.

Komaromy, M., K. Grumbach, M. Drake, K. Vranizan, N. Lurie, D. Keane, and A. Bindman. 1996. "The Role of Black and Hispanic Physicians in Providing Health Care for Underserved Populations." *New England Journal of Medicine* 334:1305–10.

Knowles, J. M. 1973. "The Hospital." *Scientific American* 229:128–38.

Leaf, A. 1978. "Health Manpower Needs." *New England Journal of Medicine* 298:1253–55.

Levit, E., M. Sabshin, et al. 1974. "Trends in Graduate Medical Education and Specialty Certification: A Tracking Study of United States Medical Graduates." *New England Journal of Medicine* 290:545–49.

Libby, D., Z. Zhou, and D. Kindig. 1997. "Will Minority Physician Supply Meet U.S. Demands?" *Health Affairs,* July–August, 205–14.

Loury, G. 1998. "The Hard Questions: Uneconomical." *New Republic,* June 29, 14–15.

Lucas, Christopher. 1994. *American Higher Education: A History.* New York: St. Martin's Griffin Press.

Ludmerer, K. 1999. *Time to Heal: American Medical Education from the Turn of the Century to the Era of Managed Care.* New York: Oxford University Press.

Martin, B. L. 1975. *Medical School Alumni: Professional Characteristics of U.S. Physicians by Medical School and Year of Graduation.* Chicago: American Medical Association.

Massey, D. S., and N. A. Denton. 1993. *American Apartheid: Segregation and the Making of the Underclass.* Cambridge: Harvard University Press.

Maynard, A. 1978. *Surgeons to the Poor: The Harlem Hospital Story.* New York: Appleton-Century-Crofts.

Meade, L. M. 1986. *Beyond Entitlement: The Social Obligations of Citizenship.* New York: Free Press.

———, ed. 1997. *The New Paternalism: Supervisory Approaches to Poverty.* Washington, D.C.: Brookings Institution.

"Medical Education in the United States (Seventy-Sixth Annual Report) 1975–1976." 1976. *Journal of the American Medical Association* 235 (2984).

Meier, K. J., J. Stewart, and R. E. Eagland. 1989. *Race, Class, and Education: The Politics of Second-Generation Discrimination.* Madison: University of Wisconsin Press.

Miller, C. A., M. K. Moos, B. J. Kotch, M. L. Brown, and M. P. Brainard. 1981. "Role of Local Health Departments in the Delivery of Ambulatory Care." *American Journal of Public Health* 71 (supplement): 15–29.

Miringoff, M., and M. L. Miringoff. 1999. *The Social Health of The Nation: How America Is Really Doing.* New York: Oxford University Press.

"Miscellany—Segregation." 1963. *Journal of the American Medical Association* 186:35.

Morais, H. M. 1969. *The History of the Negro in Medicine.* 3d ed. New York: Publishers Company.

Morbidity and Mortality Weekly Review. 2000. CDC Surveillance Summaries, vol. 49, March 24.

Moy, E., and B. Bartman. 1995. "Physician Race and Care of Minority and Medically Indigent Patients." *Journal of the American Medical Association* 273:1515–20.

Mullan, F. 2000. "The Case for More U.S. Medical Students." *New England Journal of Medicine* 343:213–17.

Myrdal, Gunnar. 1944. *An American Dilemma: The Negro Problem and Modern Democracy.* New York: Harper.

National Association for the Advancement of Colored People, Legal Defense and Education Fund (NAACP). 1976. Brief for the NAACP as amicus curiae. *Regents of the University of California v. Bakke,* 438 U.S. 265 (1978).

National Fund for Minority Engineering Students. 1976. Brief as amicus curiae. *Regents of the University of California v. Bakke,* 438 U.S. 265 (1978).

New York Public Library African American Desk Reference. 1999. New York: John Wiley and Sons.

"New York's Policy on FMG's Assailed by AMA." 1980. *American Medical News,* December 19.

Nickens, H. W., and J. J. Cohen. 1996. "Policy Perspectives on Affirmative Action." *Journal of the American Medical Association* 275:572–74.

Odegaard, C. E. 1977. *Minorities in Medicine: From Receptive Passivity to Positive Action, 1966–76.* New York: Josiah Macy Jr. Foundation.

Olds, D., R. Cole, et al. 1997. "Long-Term Effects of Home Visitation on Maternal Life Course and Child Abuse and Neglect." *Journal of the American Medical Association* 278:637–43.

Olds, D., C. Henderson, R. Cole, J. Eckenrode, H. Kitzman, D. Luckey, L. Pettitt, K. Sidora, P. Morris, and J. Powers. 1998. "Long-Term Effects of Nurse Home Visitation on Children's Criminal and Antisocial Behavior." *Journal of the American Medical Association* 280:1238–44.

Orfield, G., and S. E. Eaton. 1996. *Dismantling Desegregation: The Quiet Reversal of Brown v. Board of Education.* New York: New Press.

Patterson, J. T. 2000. *Brown v. Board of Education: A Civil Rights Milestone and Its Troubled Legacy.* New York: Oxford University Press.

Patterson, O. 1997. *The Ordeal of Integration.* Washington, D.C.: Civitas, Counterpoint Press.

Petersdorf, R. G., K. S. Turner, H. W. Nickens, and T. Ready. 1990. "Minorities in Medicine: Past, Present, and Future." *Academic Medicine* 65:663–70.

"The Progress of Black Student Matriculations at the Nation's Highest-Ranked Colleges and Universities." 1999. *Journal of Blacks in Higher Education* 25 (autumn): 8–16.

Raphael, D. 2000. "Health Inequities in the United States: Prospects and Solutions." *Journal of Public Health Policy* 21:394–427.

Ravitch, D. 1995. *National Standards in American Education.* Washington, D.C.: Brookings Institution.

Reitzes, D. C. 1958. *Negroes and Medicine.* Cambridge: Harvard University Press.

Reynolds, R. 2000. "Dr. Louis T. Wright and the NAACP: Pioneers in Hospital Racial Integration." *American Journal of Public Health* 90:883–92.

Roback, G. A. 1975. *Physician Distribution and Medical Licensure in the United States, 1974.* Center for Health Services Research and Development, American Medical Association.

Robinson, R. 2000. *The Debt: What America Owes to Blacks.* New York: Dutton.

Rosen, J. 2001. "For Race in Class, without Merit." *New Republic,* May 14, 20–22.

Rothbart, M. 1976. "Achieving Racial Equality: An Analysis of Resistance to Social Reform." In *Toward the Elimination of Racism,* ed. P. Katz. New York: Pergamon Press.

Satcher, D. 1999. "The Initiative to Eliminate Racial and Ethnic Health Disparities Is Moving Forward." *Public Health Report* 114:283–87.

Savitt, T. L. 1978. *Medicine and Slavery.* Urbana: University of Illinois Press.

Schmidt, P. 2002. "Next Stop, Supreme Court?" *Chronicle of Higher Education,* May 24, A24–28.

Schweinhart, L., H. Barnes, and D. Weikart. 1993. *Significant Benefits: The High/Scope Project Perry Preschool Study through Age 27.* Ypsilanti, Mich.: High/Scope Press.

Selengo, J. 2001. *Chronicle of Higher Education,* April 6, A29.

Shea, S., and M. T. Fullilove. 1985. "Entry of Black and Other Minority Students into U.S. Medical Schools: Historical Perspective and Recent Trends." *New England Journal of Medicine* 313:933–40.

Shinagawa, L., and M. Lang. 1998. *Atlas of American Diversity.* Walnut Creek, Calif.: Sage.

Slater, M., and E. Iler. 1991. "A Program to Prepare Minority Students for Careers in Medicine, Science, and Other High-Level Professions." *Academic Medicine* 66:220–25.

Smedley, S., A. Stith, and A. Nelson, eds. 2002. *Unequal Treatment: Confronting Racial and Ethnic Disparities in Health Care.* Report prepared by the Institute of Medicine. Washington, D.C.: National Academy Press.

Smith, C. J., ed. 1978. *Advancing Equality of Opportunity—a Matter of Justice.* Washington, D.C.: Institute for the Study of Educational Policy, Howard University.

Smith, D. B. 1999. *Health Care Divided: Race and Healing a Nation.* Ann Arbor: University of Michigan Press.

Smith, J. O. 1987. *The Politics of Racial Inequality: A Systematic Comparative Macro-Analysis from the Colonial Period to 1970.* New York: Greenwood Press.

Solow, R. M. 1998. *Work and Welfare.* With commentaries by G. Himmelfarb, A. Lewis, G. Lowry, and J. Roemer. Princeton: Princeton University Press.

Starfield, B. 2000. "Is U.S. Health Really the Best in the World?" *Journal of the American Medical Association* 284:483–85.

Steinberg, S. 1989. *The Ethnic Myth: Race, Ethnicity, and Class in America.* 2d ed. Boston: Beacon Press.

Stewart, P. 2000. "Why Xavier Remains No. 1." *Black Issues in Higher Education,* July 19, 22–26.

Summary of GMENAC Report. 1980. *Chronicle of Higher Education,* October 6.

Swain, C. 2000. "Affirmative Action: Legislative History, Judicial Interpretations, Public Consensus." In *America Becoming: Racial Trends and Their Consequences,* ed. N. Smelser, W. Wilson, and F. Mitchel, 1:318–47. Washington, D.C.: National Academy Press.

Task Force on Graduate Medical Education, Association of American Medical Colleges. 1980. *Graduate Medical Education: Proposals for the Eighties.* Washington, D.C.: AAMC.

Thompson, T. 1974. "Curbing the Black Physician Manpower Shortage." *Journal of Medical Education* 49:944–50.

Tollett, K. 1977. *The Bakke Case.* Washington, D.C.: Institute for the Study of Educational Policy, Howard University.

Udry, J. R., N. M. Morris, and K. E. Bauman. 1976. "Changes in Women's Preference for the Racial Composition of Medical Facilities, 1969–1974." *American Journal of Public Health* 66:284–86.

U.S. Commission on Civil Rights. 1977. *Statement on Affirmative Action.* U.S. Clearinghouse Publication 54, October. Washington, D.C.: U.S. Government Printing Office.

———. 1978. *Toward Equal Educational Opportunity: Affirmative Admission Programs at Law and Medical Schools.* U.S. Clearinghouse Publication 55, June. Washington, D.C.: U.S. Government Printing Office.

U.S. Department of Commerce, Bureau of the Census. 1973. *1970 Census of Population Supplementary Report, Persons of Spanish Ancestry.* Washington, D.C.: U.S. Government Printing Office.

———. 1976. *Statistical Abstract of the United States, 1976.* Washington, D.C.: U.S. Government Printing Office.

———. 1978. *1970 Census of Population Supplementary Report, Persons of Spanish Ancestry.* Washington, D.C.: U.S. Government Printing Office.

———. 1991. *Statistical Abstract of the United States, 1991.* Washington, D.C.: U.S. Government Printing Office.

———. 1992. Census of Population and Housing, 1990. Summary Tape File 3B (MRDF). Bureau of the Census (producer), Interuniversity Consortium for Political and Social Research, University of Michigan (distributor).

———. Economics and Statistics Administration. 2001. Census 2000. September.

U.S. Department of Health and Human Services. (HHS). 1979. *Healthy People: The Surgeon General's Report on Health Promoting and Disease Prevention.* Washington, D.C.: U.S. Government Printing Office.

———. 1980. *Summary Report of the Graduate Medical Education National Advisory Committee.* Washington, D.C.: U.S. Government Printing Office.

———. 1998. "Healthy People 2000 Objectives for Black Americans: Program Review." October 26. web.health.90V/healthypeople.

———. 2001. "HHS Fact Sheet." November 19. www.hhs.gov/news.

U.S. Department of Health, Education, and Welfare (DHEW). 1974. *The Supply of Health Manpower: 1970 Profiles and Projections to 1990.* DHEW Publication No. (HRA) 75-38. Washington, D.C.: U.S. Government Printing Office.

————. 1978a. *Minorities and Women in the Health Fields: Applicants, Students, and Workers.* DHEW Publication No. (HRA) 79-22. Washington, D.C.: U.S. Government Printing Office.

————. 1978b. *Minority Medical Students.* DHEW Publication No. (HRA) 78-625. Washington, D.C.: U.S. Government Printing Office.

"Washington News." 1964. *Journal of the American Medical Association* 187:15.

Watson, W. H. 1999. *Blacks in the Profession of Medicine in the United States: Against the Odds.* New Brunswick, N.J.: Transaction Publishers.

Welch, S., and J. Grubel. 1998. *Affirmative Action and Minority Enrollments in Medical and Law Schools.* Ann Arbor: University of Michigan Press.

Wellington, J. S., and P. Montero. 1978. "Equal Educational Opportunity Programs in American Medical Schools." *Journal of Medical Education* 53:633–39.

Whitehead, M. 1992. "The Concepts and Principles of Equity and Health." *International Journal of Health Services* 22:429–45.

Williams, D. R. 1998. "African American Health: The Role of the Social Environment." *Bulletin of the New York Academy of Medicine* 75:300–321.

Williams, D. R., and T. D. Rucker. 2000. "Understanding and Addressing Racial Disparities in Healthcare." *Minority Health Today* 2:30–39.

Willie, C. V., and R. R. Edmonds, eds. 1978. *Black Colleges in America.* New York: Teachers' College Press, Columbia University.

Wohl, A. 2001. "Diversity on Trial: The Fate of Affirmative Action in Education May Soon Be Decided by the Supreme Court." *American Prospect* 12:37–39.